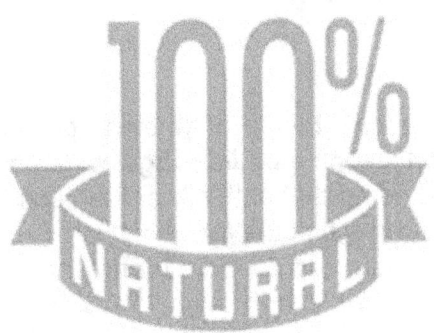

Baby

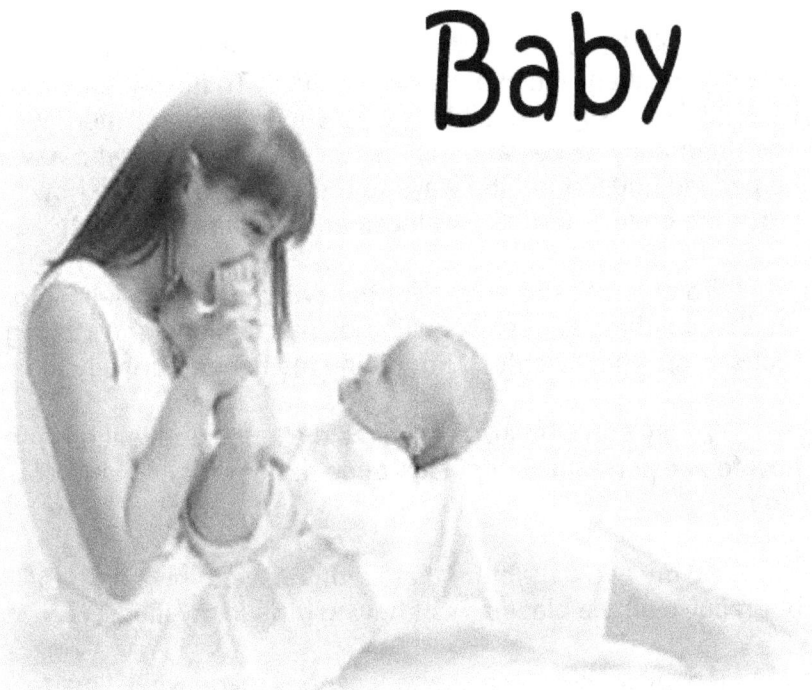

"Fertility Made Simple Plan"

-Dr. Tammy Post

Dedication

To my baby girl, Grace that I lost through the tragedy of miscarriage. I know that you are my guardian angel watching over me. I thank you for choosing that path rather than coming into this physical existence, though at the time I did not understand. You knew that you could do more for me from Heaven than on Earth. And I thank you through your loss that I now know what women go through and without that experience I would not be able to help them on their journey now.

To all those who have taught me about wellness and how to ultimately achieve it and sustain it. To the patients who have shared many difficult journeys with hormones, infertility and pregnancy losses and the mentors and coaches who have helped me understand the ways of the human body and how to crack the code of fertility, wellness and sustainable health.

To my husband, Bryan for believing in me and teaching me that anything is possible with positive thinking and staying focused on what I wanted. For loving me unconditionally.

To my son who always makes me laugh and teaches me how to see perpetually that God does things "for me" and not "to me".

To my two daughters that I didn't have to give birth to but receive all the blessings of having girls in my life.

To my family for the sacrifices they made while I made this trek and for supporting me in every way.

God who created me perfectly to share this message with the world and works with me constantly to grow into what he created me to be.

For Information about permissions to reproduce selections from this book or to purchase copies for educational, business or sales promotional use, contact:

Project Wellness
1400 SE Walton Suite 28
Bentonville, AR 72712
479-657-6800

First Edition

Printed in the USA

Table of Contents

Introduction: By Allison C.

I was diagnosed with PCOS 6 years ago. After 4 years of trying to conceive, including 3 miscarriages we tried fertility treatments. I was told my eggs were too old. We quit trying and decided I needed to just be as healthy as I could. I decided to look into Dr. Tammy.

When I met her she looked at me and said, "So, you want to have a baby!"...I began crying because that is not what I was there for and I was trying to leave it behind. She told me that she believed that I would be pregnant within a year. Dr. Tammy taught me about how my hormones accompanied with food sensitivities were making me sick. I also learned about how blood sugar in the body effects the production of hormones.

I felt so much better once I started her program. I even lost some weight which I had struggled with for years. Best of all I found out that I was pregnant again! Our baby girl was born in July and we are so thankful! I believe the tools Dr. Tammy taught me helped heal my body from the inside out and helped me conceive and carry a pregnancy to term.

My Story

I am a board certified physician, author, speaker and expert in bio-identical hormones. You may be thinking, "she's a doctor, and that's great she knows a lot, but what does she know about MY struggles".

Well I have lived many struggles including infertility. I started out with terrible menstrual cycles at a young age, was diagnosed with PCOS (polycystic ovarian syndrome) and endometriosis as well as adenomyosis (conditions that cause terrible irregular bleeding, that eventually lead to a hysterectomy, going on synthetic hormones and gaining 80 pounds and my husband and I tried for 13 years to have a baby.

During that time I did get pregnant once and had a miscarriage. Everyone knows that miscarriages are a terrible experience. But if you have never had one then it's almost impossible to understand how extremely painful both physically and emotionally they can be.

Have you or someone you know ever suffered one of the worst consequences of hormonal imbalances? Maybe you have dreamed of having a baby only to be told it's not possible. Maybe you have had complications from your periods. Maybe throughout all of this you may have from time to time blamed yourself. I know first hand that hormonal problems for women are not just "moodiness" or "unpredictable periods". They control you. Disrupt your life. Create uncertainty that you are ok and sometimes you even question if you might die from the pain of a terrible menstrual cycle. Maybe you have been to doctors that made you feel like you were crazy because your suffering seemed so out of proportion to someone who simply cannot understand.

For me it was not the painful heavy periods or the uncertainty of when I would have a cycle at all. The worst was not the ovarian cyst ruptures, endometriosis complications or even my eventual

The worst was not the infertility that I struggled with for thirteen years. The worst was the loss of my little girl.

When I was in my fourth year of medical school I got pregnant. I was about 10 weeks along when I realized I was pregnant because my periods had been so irregular. I had one of the greatest senses of peace in my entire life during that time. I was a little nervous, I longed for a little girl, I dreamed of pink bows and pretty dresses, tea parties and playing Barbie dolls with her. I had saved all my dolls from childhood just for her eventual arrival.

I stood in the small sterile apartment bathroom shaking. Barely enough room on the small sink to balance the pregnancy strip as I laid it dripping with urine precariously. I watched as the urine seeped slowly up the wand into the window of soft velvety paper. It teased and stopped, flowed and stopped, crept like fingers up the strip. It seemed an eternity until it soaked into the first space. The control. It slowly turned pink, as it should. I sighed and waited as it seeped further. My fate in the liquid penetrating the atmosphere. "What would it be?" I knew what it would be. There was no doubt. It was a feeling as sure as I knew the date and time. I had dreamed of her for years and knew this was our time. And there it was. PINK! The second line was pinkly positive!

I was immeasurably blissful for the days that followed. I told everyone I knew. I would sheepishly present myself and then explode with the news. "She's coming!" I would announce. "Gracie is coming!" I had named her long ago in a dream. I felt purpose and in touch with the universe. As the tiny ball of cells doubled, made a heart, a brain… a face, formed hands and feet… I waited. For 3 months I waited.

My mother came to visit. Drove sixteen hours from my home town to bring me a little pink outfit. She was so excited that Gracie was coming. We would wait the long wait for her and then celebrate her like my mother had celebrated me coming into this world, and love her perfect creative genius coming into physical form to make all our lives amazing. More amazing than we could ever imagine.

Then in the middle of the night. While the world slept. Grace's light went out. I went to the bathroom to urinate and wiped red. My heart stopped. Nothingness engulfed me.
I screamed into the night. I slammed the toilet tissue against the wall. Blood slinging, and waited.

I looked between my legs into the red water below to see the worst. A tiny intricate human form, I could see her heart, wispy transparent yet distinct, wrapped in what appeared to look like grapes. I collapsed on the floor and sobbed. I wrapped my arms around the toilet bowl and begged her from my soul not to leave. I waited and watched the bowl of red for an eternity until my husband arrived and flushed the toilet. My funeral - a toilet. My mourning no more than an obscene little bathroom.

I crawled to the shower, cleaned myself up, black blood caked to my legs like dried chocolate. I don't know how I made it to bed. I didn't get out of it for three days. Well-meaning people came and called. Said horrific things like, "It's for the best, or God's will. You wouldn't have wanted a baby that had something wrong with it." And worse yet, "You'll have another one."

"Oh, God, there would never be another Grace. You mean crazy woman!" I would scream inside, or something worse, but hold it in. I could not imagine how their words could sting so much. Trying to make me feel better they only crushed my soul further. The lesson I suppose to this day I have understood the value of just saying, "I'm sorry you're hurting. I'm here for you." When someone suffers tragedy. There is no way you can understand if you have never gone through that, no way it can be made better. You just have to love them in that space and comfort their soul. I also know that you can never take someone's pain away. You have to let them have it. Even if it makes you uncomfortable.

Men always want to fix things and my husband didn't know how to fix this. He was hurting and didn't want me to hurt. He told me to stop crying. Get out of bed and face the world. His inability to process my pain made him just want my feelings to go away.

The day she died... our marriage did too. Oh, we continued it on for 13 more years in an empty shell but I know that I lost two people and   maybe three that day, including part of me.

Eventually I crawled out of my zombie state. Went back to my medical school rotations. Everywhere I saw young mothers, some were alcoholics and drug addicts. In my mind unworthy of their precious gifts. I had wanted my baby so desperately and I had nothing. I felt so cheated and alone.

This is what I wrote for her all those years ago:

In the middle of the night
I knew you would never be
The life I held inside was fleeting
Faster than I could follow
Though I wanted to try
Did I ask too much?
A chance to touch a bit of heaven?
But you were not to be
And though each of us is known before we're born
You will never know how much your missed
How much you would have been kissed
The feeling of your first step
dolls, lipstick, tea parties, or the prom
College or marriage
But you will be blessed
Never to know the painful word...
Miscarriage

So, I understand the terror and the pain. Not just the physical, but the emotional... of the loss of a life that is only yours briefly, but loved so much.

If you have suffered from miscarriages or infertility, hormone imbalance of any kind, I understand and feel your pain. The struggle has helped me to understand what other's go through. I truly believe that God allows things to happen "for us" and not "to us". We learn and we guide.

Through my challenges I have learned to help women with infertility, avoid the terrible events of miscarriages and hormonal imbalance issues.

I have a deep understanding of what you may be going through and I truly want to help you.

Through our proven supplements and programs we can help balance your hormones and help with fertility in a natural way as well as regulate periods and help you regain your life and relationships.

I wish I had known then what I know now or that there had been someone to help me with my issues. I know that my journey was not in vane but to one day help others just like you… struggling and scared.

It is my honor and privilege to be that voice today for so many.

Chapter One

So you want a baby?

More importantly` your baby wants you. Somewhere out there is your precious soul just waiting to come into your life. Just think, scientists speculate that the odds of you yourself being born and existing as you today, are at about one in 400 trillion ($4x10^{14}$). Yet, given those odds, you are here. I believe that when we are meant to be here, we arrive. Your baby is out there just waiting to be born. So why is it so hard? Why are you struggling to welcome your precious soul that is in line ready and eager to come into your life?

Given that you are here and serving your higher purpose I have no doubt in my mind that your little bundle of joy is just an extension of you. There may have been great odds of you coming into existence and being born but now that you are here, your baby is just an extension of you.

Why do you want a baby? They are amazing of course. I remember all the years wanting a baby; thirteen to be exact. I would imagine how my baby would feel pressed against my skin. Sometimes in the department store I would smell the baby lotion, and let the simple fragrance envelop me. I dreamed of snuggling my baby and how it would feel to hear the words, "Mom, Mamma, or Mommy" one day.

A child is a special relationship. You have a special bond. A child will love you unconditionally. You can be the worst parent in the world and your child will still love you. We as humans crave that type of love.

I have heard it said that there are three types of love. The love that God has for us which we cannot begin to understand. The love we have for a spouse or significant other, but even that love often feels somewhat conditional…We want that other person to behave a certain way or we are challenged in our "Do they really love me?" Lastly there is the love that we have with our children. They can misbehave or disappoint us and we always love them, just like they will always love you.

It is in our DNA to reproduce. Our hormones drive our desires on so many levels from the very act of lovemaking to the need to nurture and be nurtured.

Yet here you are struggling, or maybe you have a loved one that is struggling to have a baby. Given the technology in today's world it seems that we should not have any trouble with fertility. It's true that we have come a long way with technology. We have designer drugs and in the lab we can grow a baby in a petri dish.

Medicine has evolved, scientists have completed extensive research, and now we have fancy procedures like IVF (in vitro fertilization) and can freeze sperm. But the simple truth of the matter is the basic science of fertility is often hidden from the general public, and even from doctors. They didn't teach me this stuff in medical school. Why?...I don't know. I have many reasons to think that big pharma has every reason to keep you struggling so that you will buy expensive medications and keep hoping. The physiology is very simple. The truth has always been right there all along, and I'm going to share the simple truth with you and what you can do about it.

You want a baby? It's a simple matter of understanding how it works. I think we all know how you get pregnant, but what is the process leading up to you getting pregnant, or the things that might be interfering physiologically that interfere with the conception process that you may not be aware of.

In my research on the internet all that I have been able surmise is there are either one of two paths. Going to a fertility specialist and the associated complicated testing and procedures, taking dangerous medications and more; or the "natural" ways are presented as "lose weight" and get healthy. But if you choose the "natural" path there is a lot of Information that is missing and this simple plan will tell you what you need to know that until now has not been shared with you in in a simple and easy to follow, organized path.

If you have struggled for a month or many years, right now I want you to take a deep breath and relax. The answers are so simple you'll   probably get angry that no one shared this information with you before.

If you have blamed yourself? Again, I want you to take a deep breath and relax. It most likely has nothing to do with you or anything you have done wrong (or at least knew about) and it is my goal to make it very   simple for you.

Given the confusing information you have received and misinformation that is widely available and even more troublesome distributed; it's a wonder any of us have ever had a baby at least in the past four to six decades. There is so much going on in our environment it's a miracle when we do get pregnant and that we don't have a plethora of birth defects to deal with. The reality of the matter is that we do…In the U.S. about one in every 33 babies (3%) are born with a birth defect and birth defects are one of the leading causes of infant death accounting for more than 20% of all infant deaths according to the Centers for Disease Control. This is not meant to scare you, but to educate you so that you when you start down the path of completing this plan and get pregnant you do not have to deal with the tragedy of losing what you worked so hard to achieve… your treasured "healthy" baby.

We are going to clear the smoke and take aim at all this confusion. In fact I'm going to nail it down to a simple, easy to follow process that will have that baby in your arms in no time. I have never had a patient fail to achieve pregnancy while following my system. It ALWAYS works as long as dad is healthy and you don't have any major structural abnormalities (like you don't have a uterus, or have a major illness, etc.)!

There will be some work involved. I said it was simple, I didn't say it was easy. But if you really want that precious baby and you want that   baby to be 100% natural, without dangerous drugs and procedures then let's get to work.

If you are struggling to get pregnant then there is something wrong with your underlying female health. We have to get you healthy so you can achieve a successful pregnancy. The environment has many issues that may be at play working against you, that are affecting your hormones and your ability to get pregnant. Once we clear this smoke you can start making choices that you never knew you needed to make before. More importantly these are changes that will keep you healthy in a sustainable way.

The basics of the plan are as follows:

1. You need to understand what environmental issues influence your health, that they are not your fault, and what you can do to take back your health

2. You need to understand how hormones work to maximize your efforts

3. You must educate yourself about nutrients that will not only allow you to get pregnant, maintain a healthy pregnancy, and have a healthy baby; but keep you healthy after childbirth and for the rest of your life so you can feel good and be a great parent, grandparent and great-grandparent!

Chapter Two

The Cost of Infertility Treatment –Not What You Think

I'm going to share some statistics with you but these statistics do not take into account the stress and anxiety that you may experience while trying achieve a successful conception. The more you worry the more stress you have. Each menstrual cycle creates more fear and anxiety when it doesn't happen. Each home pregnancy test that you take that is negative creates more of that anxiety. "Maybe I'll never have a baby", you start to think and then you start blaming yourself and the guilt and shame cycle consumes you.

These statistics show that you are not alone. But I know that doesn't make you feel any better.

- **6.7 Million women ages 15-44 have impaired fertility (ability to get pregnant or carry a baby to term)**

- **10.9% of women ages 15-44 have impaired fertility**

- **1.5 million married women ages 15-44 are infertile (unable to get pregnant after at least 12 consecutive months of unprotected sex with their husband)**

- **6% of married women ages 15-44 are diagnosed <u>infertile</u>**

- **7.4 million women ages 15-44 have sought infertility services**

- **1 in 6 American couples have trouble getting pregnant**

  (Source: National Survey of Family Growth, Centers for Disease Control and Prevention [CDC] 2006-2010).

Infertility is NOT an inconvenience; it is a severe emotional and physical crisis in the families that if affects.

Lets take a look at some of the financial costs of infertility. We can break this down into national costs and personal costs.

National Costs:

- **Infertility is an estimated $2 billion industry annually in the United States**

- **Pharmaceutical companies are investing millions in fertility-related drugs.**

- **Clinic management corporations traded on Wall Street are in the business of making a profit on infertility treatment for I investors. Brokers are charging fees to help couples find egg donors and surrogate mothers.**

- **The number of U.S. clinics offering IVF has been racing upward since the mid-1980s, to about 330 today.**

And the personal potential financial costs:

The cost for fertility treatments and fertility drugs are a significant concern for many couples struggling with infertility. Infertility and IVF insurance coverage is not common and a lot of variation is seen in what is covered and what is left for the patient to pay. The average cost of in vitro fertilization in the U.S. is currently about $11,000 to $12,000 and this does not include the medications or lab testing. This is per "try". If you try multiple times or want more than one baby, some couples can spend over *$100,000 trying* to have a family.

If you go the "assisted reproductive technologies (ART)" route most are not covered by insurance, the patient has to pay "out-of-pocket," often leading to increased stress as well as long-term financial burdens.

The American Society of Reproductive Medicine (ASRM) lists the average price of an in vitro fertilization (IVF) cycle in the U.S. to be $12,400 Here is the raw reality of what trying to have a family may cost using medical intervention.

•Average cost of an IUI (intrauterine insemination) cycle: $865; Median Cost: $350

•Average Cost of an IVF (in vitro fertilization) cycle using fresh embryos (not including medications): $8,158; Median Cost: $7,500- Medications for IVF are $3,000 $5,000 per fresh cycle on average

•Average additional cost of ICSI (intra-cytoplasmic sperm injection) procedure: $1,544; Median Cost: $1,500

•Average additional cost of PGD (pre-implantation genetic diagnosis) procedure: $3,550; Median Cost: $3,200

Chapter Three

Getting Healthy For Your Baby

Let's start with a simple quiz:

Take this 10 question quiz to evaluate for any issues that you may have.

1. How old are you?

Choose one

I am under 25 years old

I am between 25 and 29 years old

I am between 30 and 34 years old

I am between 35 and 39 years old

I am 40+ years old

2. How long have you been trying to get pregnant?

Choose one

Under 3 months

Under 6 months

6-12 months

Over 12 months

Over 2 years

3. Are your menstrual periods irregular or do you miss periods?

Choose one

I have regular periods every 26-28 days

My periods are about every 2 weeks

My periods are all over the place

I sometimes go 2-3 months without a period

I haven't had a period for over 6 months

4. Are your periods painful or heavy?

Choose one

My periods are light

My periods are moderate

My periods are heavy

My periods are extremely heavy (I spend a fortune on pads and tampons)

My periods are very heavy with clots and pain

5. Is your spouse healthy, has he had his testosterone checked and/or to see if sperm is adequate?

Choose one

Yes, we have had him checked out and all is ok

Yes, we have had him checked and his testosterone is low

Yes, we have had his sperm checked an it is ok

No, we have not had him checked out.

I don't know

6. Have you had any miscarriages?

Choose one

I have not had any miscarriages

I have had one miscarriage

I have had 1-3 miscarriages

I have had more than 5 miscarriages

I don't know if I have had any miscarriages or they were so early I wasn't aware

7. Do you take any medications (not for fertility) on a regular basis?

Choose one

I take no medications

I take 1 medication

I take 2-3 medications

I take 4-7 medications

I take more than 8 medications

8. Have you ever had any lab testing, ultrasound or imaging study of the female reproductive system to make sure that structurally you are capable of conceiving and maintaining a healthy pregnancy, or have you been diagnosed with endometriosis or polycystic ovarian syndrome (PCOS)?

Choose one

No I have not had any tests done

I have had an ultrasound and everything was ok

I have been diagnosed with PCOS

I have been diagnosed with endometriosis

I have problems with my tubes, ovaries or uterus

9. How often do you have intercourse?

Choose one

Every day

2-3 times a week

2-5 times during ovulation or most fertile days

2-3 times a month

Less than 2-3 times a month

10. How would you rate your stress level?

Choose one

I don't think I am stressed at all

Very little stress (other than worried about infertility)

Moderate life stress (work, home, family issues)

Moderate to high stress

Very high stress (I don't think I can cope with life most days)

So let's look at the major reasons that you might have trouble getting pregnant.

- 25% of infertile couples have more than one factor that contributes to their infertility.

- Irregular or abnormal ovulation accounts for approximately 25 percent of all female infertility problems.

- Most couples (80-90%) resort to treating with conventional medical therapies such as medication or surgery. The good news is it can be treated **naturally**, safely and effectively!

What areas do you need to look at for "getting healthy"? Well let's look at some statistics on what might interfere with your getting pregnant.

Twelve percent of all infertility cases are a result of the woman either weighing too little or too much. It is possible for women with body weight disorders to reverse their infertility by attaining and maintaining a healthy weight.

Men and Women who smoke have decreased fertility.
The risk of miscarriage is higher for pregnant women who smoke.
Up to 13 percent of female infertility is caused by cigarette smoking. Lastly, STD's like a Chlamydia infection if left untreated, can cause infertility.

What is optimal for getting pregnant?

- Between 25 and 29 years of age is the optimal time for fertility as long as you ovulate normally, have healthy menstrual cycles and your partner has a good sperm count. If you are 35 or older it may be more difficult to get pregnant.

- It is recommended that your BMI be less than 27 but not less than 23 and 22% body fat is optimal

- Not having any history of miscarriages. Having 3 or more miscarriages in a row makes it more difficult to get pregnant and may mean that you need to be assessed for MTHFR a genetic defect of the metabolism or methylation of a B-vitamin called folate and this could lead to birth defects if you successfully conceive. But rest assured we have that covered. Taking Methyl-folate will dramatically reduce your risk of future miscarriage and birth defects in your baby.

- Not having any other medical issues. Having other medical issues or taking medications may need to be addressed before attempting to conceive.

- Low Stress level. High stress can cause excess cortisol levels and affect your ability to conceive.

- Making love 2-3 times during your fertile time (ovulation) is optimal

The Root of hormone issues

It's not your fault...

Most issues with fertility are from having hormone imbalance. Having spent the past 15 years trying to understand how hormones affect every part of the body, mostly in attempt to help myself and the symptoms I suffered, I now have an expert level understanding of what is going on. I have helped thousands of women with hormone imbalance issues.

I want to share with you some of the changes that have happened to us over the past four to six decades that have led to our hormones having trouble with balance.

Hormones are chemical messengers in our body that direct every process that occurs. You name it. A hormone is responsible for directing the traffic. Sleep. Cholesterol production. Metabolism. Hunger. Feeling full. Feeling happy. Sex drive.... And the list goes on and on.

So getting your hormones balanced is the first step!

When your hormones are balanced you are more likely to have a healthy body weight for getting pregnant and the bottom line is that the female/male reproductive hormones must be in alignment for you to get pregnant!

I believe the first place we have to look for hormone imbalance is a most unlikely place that you may have never thought of...

THE GUT!!!...and by gut I mean the intestines... This is not only what we eat but how well we absorb the nutrients from what we eat.

How did our intestines or gut get so out of balance????

Well there are lots of reasons. Let's break them down one by one.

1. People are eating more junk food than ever before. From the 1940's to today our eating out fast food has increased by over 40%.

2. Sugar consumption has sky rocketed.

Source: Johnson RJ, et al. Potential role of sugar (fructose) in the epidemic of hypertension, obesity and the metabolic syndrome, diabetes, kidney disease, and cardiovascular disease. The American Journal of Clinical Nutrition, 2007.

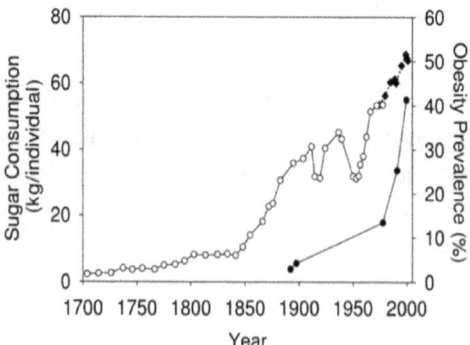

Added sugar is the single **worst** ingredient in the modern diet.
Numerous studies show that eating excess amounts of added sugar
can have harmful effects on metabolism, leading to insulin resistance,
belly fat gain, high triglycerides and small, dense LDL cholesterol...
to name a few, It also has adverse effects on hormones related to
obesity.

Its no surprise that, studies show that people who eat
the most sugar are at a high risk of future weight gain and obesity.

In the 1970's we started with the "Low Fat" craze thinking that
fat in our diet was making us "fat". Our true obesity epidemic started
in our country at that time.

Why all the sugar? Why did we start consuming more?

3. Low Fat Diet Fads

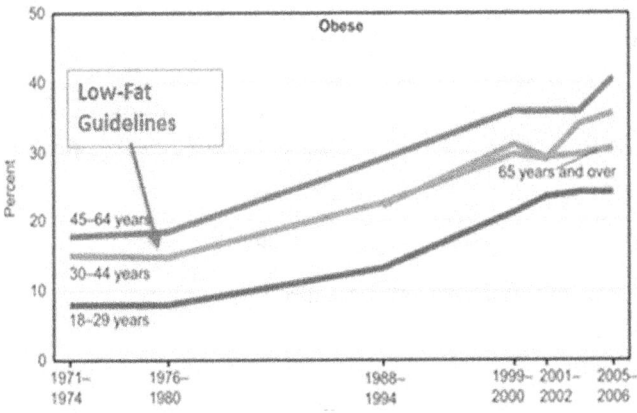

Source: National Center for Health Statistics (US). Health, United States, 2008: With Special
Feature on the Health of Young Adults. 2009 Mar. Chartbook.

When people aren't eating fat, what do they eat??? Sugar! And lots of it. Low fat foods must use something to make it taste better and that is usually chemicals like MSG, more salt or sugar. Putting the emphasis on fat, while giving processed low-fat foods high in sugar - a free pass, may have contributed to negative changes in the population's diet. There are also massive long-term studies showing that the low-fat diet does NOT cause weight loss, and does not prevent heart disease or cancer.

4. We eat more on the holidays

Most people don't gain weight overnight... it happens slowly, over years and decades. But the rate is uneven throughout the year and spikes **dramatically** during the holidays, a time when people tend to binge on all sorts of delicious holiday foods and eat much more than their bodies need.

The problem is that sometimes people don't lose all the weight back. They might gain 3 pounds, but only lose 2 after the holidays are over, leading to slow and steady weight gain over time. Yo-yo diets lead to what I call "dieting with interest". Every time you lose a few pounds by starving yourself or cutting calories you up regulate the hormone that are protective for us and cause us to hold more fat. In fact, a large percentage of   people's lifetime weight gain can be explained *just* by the 6 week holiday period.

5. Junk food is cheaper

One factor that has most likely contributed to increased consumption is a lower price of food. Food prices have dropped in the past 40 years. But we are eating more junk and processed foods. Healthy food isn't cheap...processed food is cheap. In fact, real foods are so expensive that a lot of people can't even afford them. How are those less fortunate supposed to stand a chance if the only food they can afford (and access) is highly processed junk, high in sugar, refined grains and added oils?

6. People are drinking their calories

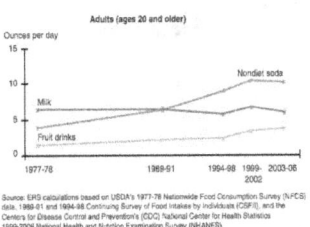

Adults (ages 20 and older)

Ounces per day

Nondiet soda

Milk

Fruit drinks

1977-78   1989-91   1994-98 1999- 2003-06
                                2002

Source: ERS calculations based on USDA's 1977-78 Nationwide Food Consumption Survey (NFCS) data, 1989-91 and 1994-98 Continuing Survey of Food Intakes by Individuals (CSFII), and the Centers for Disease Control and Prevention's (CDC) National Center for Health Statistics 1999-2006 National Health and Nutrition Examination Survey (NHANES).

We were never meant to drink our calories. Our ancestors certainly didn't. The brain is the main organ in charge of regulating our energy balance... making sure that we don't starve and don't accumulate excess fat. Well, it turns out that the brain doesn't "register" liquid sugar calories in the same way as it does solid calories. So if you consume a certain number of calories from a sugary drink, then your brain doesn't automatically make you eat fewer calories of something else instead. Fruit juices are no better and have similar amounts of sugar as soft drinks. Studies have shown that a *single* daily serving of a sugar-sweetened beverage is linked to a 60.1% increased risk of obesity in children. Sugar is bad... but sugar in liquid form is even worse.

7. We sit behind a desk all day

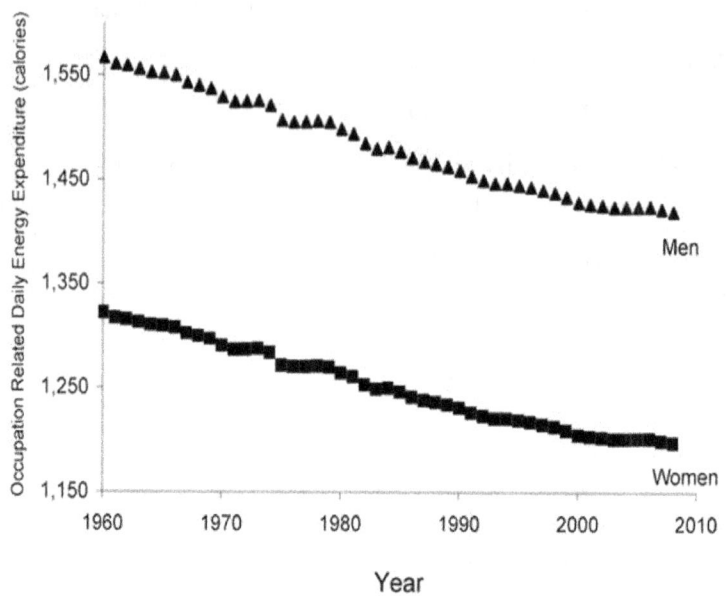

Source: Church TS, et al. Trends over 5 Decades in U.S. Occupation-Related Physical Activity and Their Associations with Obesity. Plus One, 2011.

We spend more time on the computer and behind a desk than decades ago. We're just burning fewer calories than we used to. Although leisure time physical activity (exercise) has increased, it is also true that people now have jobs that are less physically demanding. The graph above shows how people are now burning around 100 fewer calories per day in their jobs, which may contribute to weight gain over time.

8. We eat more with friends and on the weekends

Who do you eat with? And when?

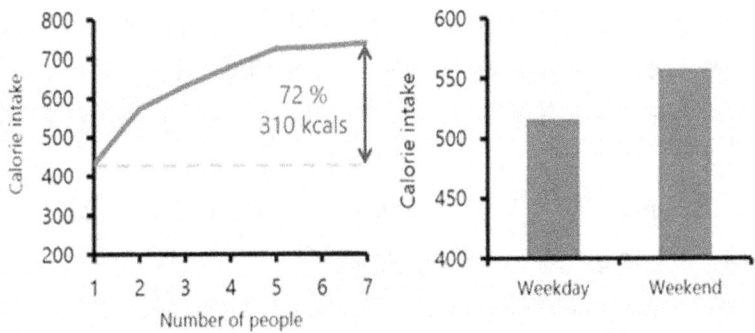

Source: Dr. Stephan Guyenet. Why do we Overeat? A Neurobiological Perspective. 2014.

The social environment is another factor that determines calorie intake. For example, eating in a group can dramatically increase the number of calories consumed. According to one paper, eating a meal with several people can increase calorie intake by **up to 72%**, or 310 calories in a single meal. There are also studies showing that people tend to eat more during weekends.

9. We don't sleep enough

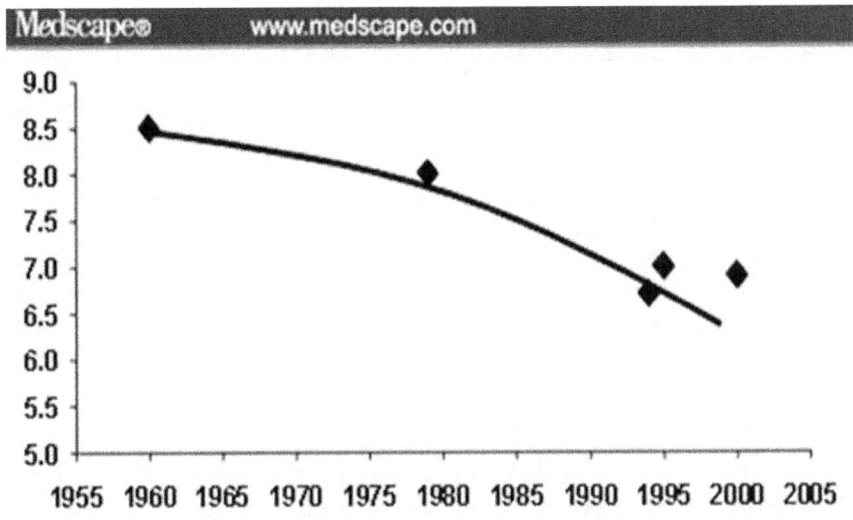

Source: Cauter EV, et al. The Impact of Sleep Deprivation on Hormones and Metabolism. Medscape, 2005.

Sleep regulates a hormone called leptin. Leptin is a hormone that regulates fat and makes us feel "not hungry". Americans are simply sleeping less.

Sleep is often overlooked when it comes to weight gain and obesity. Sleep quality is important too. The television show the biggest loser always does a pre-participation physical and checks for sleep issues like sleep apnea because they know that the likelihood of losing weight is diminished if the participants have a sleep disorder. It is scientifically proven that poor sleep has negative effects on various hormones (especially   leptin) that are related to weight gain, and can contribute to increased   hunger and cravings.

In recent decades, average sleep duration has decreased by 1-2 hours per night. The reasons for this are numerous, but increased artificial lighting and electronics are likely contributors. It turns out, short sleep   duration is one of the **strongest** individual risk factors for obesity. It is linked to an 89% increased risk in children, and a 55% increased risk in adults.

10. We are consuming more calories

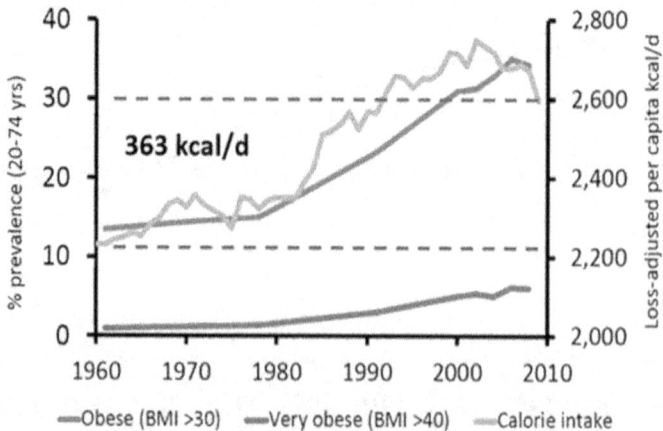

—Obese (BMI >30)   —Very obese (BMI >40)   —Calorie intake

Source: Dr. Stephan Guyenet. Why Do We Overeat? A Neurobiological Perspective.2014. (Data from CDC NHANES surveys and USDA food disappearance data)

We are eating more calories than we did in the past decades. Just look at a bucket of popcorn at the movies. It's huge and pizza slices are larger, and then SUPERSIZE me please (not!)

20 years ago a hamburger had approximately 333 calories, today on average 590 calories (that's 257 more calories). A slice of pizza 20 years ago on average was 500 calories, today a slice on average has 850. This increase in calorie consumption alone is enough to account for our obesity epidemic.

11. Toxins in our environment

I have shared with patients for years that I suspected pesticides are dangerous but didn't really realize the full extent. I know that certain pesticides resemble estrogen in the body (we call these Xeno-estrogens) they can cause hormone irregularities. I also found that certain chemicals that may be found in "Round-Up" as an example disrupt our digestive tracts leading to a leaky gut that I will discuss at length as you read on.

I have seen a rise in gluten intolerance in food sensitivity testing and knew that it was very problematic for healthy digestion but recently learned that there is something going on with the wheat supply that is not well known by the public.

The issues with our wheat supply go beyond gluten or hybridization, genetically modified or the organic versus non-organic hype, but the   problem actually lies in the pesticides used on the wheat. Gluten and wheat hybrids have been consumed for many, many years and have not caused widespread problems. So why all the problems with gluten and wheat now? It's the pesticides!

Standard wheat harvest protocol in the U.S. is to saturate the wheat fields with "Round Up" several days before the mechanical combine   harvesters harvest the fields to allow for easier and larger harvest as dead withered wheat is easier to plow. "Round Up" is routinely used by all wheat growers in the U.S. and contains the deadly active ingredient glyphosate which affects our gastrointestinal absorptive abilities and blocks essential pathways in our livers to clear other toxins we are exposed to. It also disrupts all the pathways found in beneficial intestinal microbes which are critical for us to able to process, synthesize and absorb critical amino acids and nutrients. Friendly gut bacteria, also called probiotics play a crucial role in all of our digestive processes. Lack of these lead to being essentially malnourished.

Glyphosate exposure is slow and insidious over months and years as inflammation gradually gains a foothold in the cellular systems of the body. The consequences of this systemic Inflammation are most may include:

- Gastrointestinal disorders

- Obesity

- Diabetes

- Heart Disease

- Depression

- Autism

- Infertility

- Cancer

- Multiple Sclerosis

Alzheimer's disease

And the list goes on and on and on …

Even if you think you have no trouble digesting wheat, it is still very wise to avoid conventional wheat as much as possible in your diet! The bottom line is that avoidance of conventional wheat in the United States is absolutely imperative even if you don't currently have a gluten allergy or wheat sensitivity. The increase in the amount of glyphosate applied to wheat closely correlates with the rise of celiac disease and gluten intolerance.

These diseases are not just genetic in nature, but also have an environmental cause as not all patient symptoms are alleviated by eliminating gluten from the diet. The effects of deadly glyphosate on your biology are so insidious that lack of symptoms today means literally nothing. If you don't have problems with wheat now, you will in the future if you keep eating conventionally produced, toxic wheat!

Obviously, if you've already developed a sensitivity or allergy to wheat, you must avoid it..Period!

Ok so what do we do about all this?...We may have known all this but what do we do now? and "how does it apply to me?" you may be asking.

First what I am asking you to do is to simply be aware of what has happened in our country over the past four-six decades that are influencing our environment. This awareness will help you see that you have been duped.

TAKE A DEEP BREATH! AND RELAX!

After you realize that you are not to blame and what has influences you then you can begin to take simple action. We will nail this down to a few simple things that you can do to start changing your life and reclaiming your balance.

It is important to keep in mind that it is not some collective moral failure that drives our obesity. All behavior is driven by the underlying biology... and the way the diet and environment have changed has altered the way our brains and hormones work. In other words, these changes have caused malfunctions in the biological systems that are supposed to prevent us from getting fat or getting pregnant.

This is the underlying reason for the increased calorie intake and weight gain, NOT a lack of willpower, as some people would have you believe.

So where do we go from here?

Get out a pen and start writing these simple steps down.

1. Get some lab work done to see how out of balance you are, this should include

Vitamin D, Vitamin B12, iron, kidney and liver testing
Full hormone panel (estradiol, estrone, estriol, testosterone, DHEA, cortisol, and a full thyroid panel)
Food sensitivity testing

2. Eat out less and limit "junk food"
3. Decrease sugar consumption (read labels as sugar is hidden in everything) if it appears first on a label then it is the MAIN ingredient, BEWARE!

4. Don't concentrate on "Low FAT"- low fat means more preservative and more SUGAR

5. Be aware of Holidays and have a strategy for not binging

6. Be aware that junk food is cheap and make better choices

7. Never drink your calories (water only!)

8. If you work a desk job, especially long hours get up and move, take a walk on your lunch break, and get into a regular exercise routine after work

9. Be mindful that when you eat with others you are likely to eat more and watch out for weekend splurges on calories and treats

10. Make an effort to get 6-8 hours of sleep a night. If you aren't sleeping well get your hormones balanced.

11. Consume less calories, be aware of portion distortion

12. Don't eat wheat from the U.S. and eat organic pesticide free as much as possible and avoid gluten if at all possible as most people have developed intolerance at this point.

Just being aware that so much has insidiously affected you should make you realize that you are not to blame. Subconscious habits are at play and our environment is making you sick and possibly fat or malnourished and infertile.

A few simple choices can be a game changer...

One more thing that I want to mention is some of the fortification processes that have been implemented and un-implemented. For example iodine, which is primarily necessary for healthy thyroid function was found to be deficient several decades ago and so fortification of this went into the salt supply. You can only imagine what issues this can bring up. Then there is folate, a vital B-vitamin in every cellular process in the body. I will go into this in more detail on folate metabolism and preventing birth defects.

It was found that as we started eating more junk food and less vegetables that the incidence of spina bifida (a neural tube defect) in newborns increased. Fortification was noted to be necessary to prevent this but folate was expensive to extract so fortification was made with folic acid which is cheaper to produce. However if you have a genetic defect called MTHFR (methyl tetrahydrofolate reductase) the enzyme need to break down folic acid and can't do this properly you can accumulate homocysteine. More on that later about fertility and health babies...

So what to eat????...

- Why understand this?

- How do you know you have food sensitivities?

- What is leaky gut?

- How to get started even before you have a blood test...8 trigger foods

- Food allergy testing

- Detoxification

Why understand nutrition? Nutrition is just one pillar of a full comprehensive design for overall health and metabolic well-being but it is an essential pillar. Without any one pillar the roof will fall. We must begin to think in terms of food not as a social engagement but something that sustains life. EAT TO LIVE! Food is eaten to sustain life, provide energy, and promote growth and repair of tissues.

Macmillan Dictionary

So, what if you are eating "HEALTHY"????

Well most people are eating "healthy" things they don't even know are literally making them fat or indirectly or directly infertile. We had a movement in our country a few years ago to go "FAT FREE". We thought simply that "FAT" in foods must make us "FAT". Worse yet we thought that the fat in foods was causing cholesterol or fat in the blood and therefore heart and blood vessel issues leading to stroke and cardiovascular disease. We found that this wasn't true at all.

When people stopped eating a lot of fat, do you know what they ate more of???????? SUGAR!!!!!

We found that there was more obesity and more heart disease than ever. The sugar caused inflammation through insulin resistance and cortisol increases and adrenal exhaustion. We saw an increase in belly fat and diabetes. We were clearly very wrong.

So if that wasn't the answer then what is? I have patients who try to decrease sugar or carbs and still gain weight or can't lose weight. Well I stumbled on to a very straightforward and interesting way to eat which is the basis for sustainable weight loss and wellness forever. Want to hear about it? Of course you do or you wouldn't be reading this.

Well there are foods that you may consider healthy but may not be right for you. "But how do I know????"

You probably don't know. But I will tell you not knowing is hurting you. Let me go into an analogy that one of our coaches shared with me.

Imagine you have a car and you have no idea what kind of gas it takes. You go to the pump and you look at the unleaded pump and the diesel fuel pump. Which one do you use? What if you guess and you are wrong? How far will your car go? If you put the wrong fuel in what will be the fix? You have to have the pipes drained right? Well your body is no different. You might think certain foods are healthy but they might not be the right fuel for you. And what do you do if you have the wrong fuel in your tank??? This is the basis for understanding food sensitivities and detox.

But first, let me ask you…

Are you experiencing…….???

1. Digestive issues such as gas, bloating, diarrhea or irritable bowel syndrome (IBS)?

2. Seasonal allergies or asthma?

3. Hormonal imbalances such as menopause symptoms, heavy periods, endometriosis, PMS or PCOS? Low libido? Hot flashes?

4. Diagnosis of an autoimmune disease such as rheumatoid arthritis, Hashimoto's thyroiditis, lupus, psoriasis, or celiac disease?

5. Fatigue?

6. Chronic fatigue?

7. Fibromyalgia? Hurt all the time for no apparent reason?

8. Mood and mind issues such as depression, anxiety, attention deficit issues?

9. Skin issues such as acne, rosacea, or eczema? Itching

10. Diagnosis of yeast infections, or food allergies or intolerances?

11. Memory loss?

12. Cancer, Aging, or heart disease?

If you said yes to any of these? You probably have food sensitivities. Before we talk about food sensitivities we need to discuss a controversial topic that is very pertinent to our discussion called "Leaky Gut"!

What is..... LEAKY GUT

Normal Intestines   Leaky Intestines

Even if you ate veggies from the Garden of Eden, organic and rich with nutrients you would still have to have a perfectly healthy digestive tract, stomach and intestine, to absorb the nutrients from that food. The intestine or gut is naturally permeable to very small molecules in order to absorb these vital nutrients. In fact, regulating intestinal permeability is one of the basic functions of the cells that line the intestinal wall. In sensitive people, gluten can cause the gut cells to release "Zonulin", a protein that can break apart tight junctions in the intestinal lining. Other factors — such as infections, toxins, stress and age — can also cause these tight junctions to break apart.

Once these tight junctions are broken apart you have a leaky gut. When your gut is leaky, things like toxins, microbes, undigested food particles, and more can escape from your intestines and travel throughout your body via your bloodstream. Your immune system marks these "foreign invaders" as pathogens and attacks them.

So, what causes leaky gut?

The main culprits are toxins (pesticides) unhealthy junk foods with preservative and sugar, infections, and gluten, a protein found in wheat, and inflammatory foods like dairy, sugar (which feeds the yeast in the gut) and excessive alcohol are suspected as well. The most common infectious causes are yeast, intestinal parasites, and small intestine bacterial overgrowth. Toxins come in the form of medications, like Motrin, Advil, steroids, antibiotics, and acid-reducing drugs, and environmental toxins like mercury, pesticides and BPA from plastics. Stress, leaking stomach acid into the intestines, hormone changes and age also contribute to a leaky gut.

The good news is there's a solution to healing leaky gut. To keep it simple, here are some basics to start with…

1. Remove foods and factors that damage the gut such as sugar, grains, dairy and GMO foods, non-organic foods, acidic substances like coffee and drugs like ibuprofen, acid reducers, and non-essential antibiotics and ask your doctor about medications that you may not need. **Get food allergy testing!** Identify your specific food sensitivities and remove them from your diet. A 21 day detox protocol of eliminating the foods you are sensitive is essential to healing the gut. If your car had diesel fuel in it and it was an unleaded gas engine you would need to remove the wrong fuel from the line.

2. Replace with healing foods like Bone Broth, Fermented Vegetables and Coconut and Super seeds like chia seeds, flaxseeds, and hemp seeds (as long as they are not on your food sensitivity/allergy list). Also, consuming foods that have anti-inflammatory Omega-3 fats are beneficial such as grass-fed beef, lamb, and wild caught fish like salmon.

1. Repair with specific supplements, these include specific amino   acids, magnesium, digestive enzymes, pro-biotics and anti-inflammatories. Certain amino acids act like "gut spackling" and protects and coats the intestinal wall, and acts as an anti-inflammatory as well as does Aloe-Vera licorice, Reservatrol and Turmeric among many we recommend. Digestive enzymes ensure that food is fully digested, decreasing the chance of undigested foods traversing the leaky gut and causing immune response. Magnesium relaxes smooth muscle in the gut keeping things moving.

2. Rebalance with pro-biotics, last but most importantly this is THE Vital Part to Healing Your Gut. You must rebalance with the right probiotics. Many on the market have the wrong ratio or have Ingredients that may make your issues worse. It is essential to get at least 100 billion units the right ratio of bacteria.

       If you can follow the above protocol you are well on your way to healing your gut for good! If you don't have access to a food sensitivity test then just avoid gluten and dairy while trying to get pregnant.

Leaky Gut: The inability to absorb vital nutrients can cause imbalances in the system.

Food allergy/sensitivity testing is a vital piece to the balance that the system is seeking as well as supplements that heal the digestive process.

When I first learned about food sensitivities, I was working with a chiropractor. He was using food sensitivities for joint pain, chronic pain, fibromyalgia and all the maladies that most patients seek out a chiropractor for. I have always been amazed at how chiropractors know things that traditional doctors don't. They don't have a prescription pad at their fingertips so they have to learn what "works" if they really want to get results. He taught me the basics of how certain foods trigger inflammation in the body and this inflammation spreads to joints, muscles, and tendons causing pain but more than that this inflammation is in the blood vessels and causing more insidious disease that may end up in heart disease, strokes, cancer autoimmune disease and possible cancer. I watched as he ordered test after test and yielded amazing results.

I had a patient who came in one day with obvious hormone imbalance and terrible fibromyalgia. I was thinking it was the hormone imbalance but after that issue was corrected she still continued to have pain. So I did what my chiropractor friend recommended and ordered the food sensitivity test.

She returned for the results and I explained how it worked. She seemed skeptical and we scheduled her a three-month follow up appointment. Fast forward to that appointment. I watched her walk into the room. Without limping. Without her cane and without obvious distress. She had a glow about her that I could not explain. Her skin was brighter and her mood lighter. She took a seat and although her physical state was remarkably improved she had an energy about her that was confusing. She smiled softly. I noticed that she appeared about twenty pounds lighter than I had seen her last.

"Looks like you are doing much better!" I exclaimed.

"Oh, I am... but..."

"But what?!?" I looked puzzled.

"I am doing amazing. I have lost twenty pounds. My joints do not hurt and the muscle pain is ninety percent improved. I have followed the food sensitivity test and had remarkable results. I am quite upset, however."

"Go on..." I encouraged her.

"I am very frustrated because over six years ago, a doctor did the food sensitivity test on me and recommended that I make dietary changes. I thought he was crazy. I'm upset because I have suffered for over six years with these symptoms and the answer was so simple. Right in front of me! It took you with your confidence to convince me, or maybe just the tremendous suffering to finally take the leap and make some changes. I am so grateful for the change in my life but frustrated that I didn't listen sooner and I have suffered so much all these years."

I was amazed, and I took this experience to heart. I started using the test on everyone that I could think of with chronic pain. I never really thought about the weight loss as I thought that was just an effect of her eating less.

Fast forward a few years and many patient success stories (all the while not acknowledging the effects of the weight loss) and I had a husband and wife come in the office one day. He was having terrible gastrointestinal symptoms. His wife was very frustrated and felt that it was affecting his health. He had terrible gas, bloating, and constipation alternating with diarrhea every time he ate. He had been diagnosed with "IBS" or irritable bowel syndrome and put on many prescription medications that simply did not help. It was affecting his work, his home life and his sleep. He was in terrible pain all over and his hormones were all out of balance as indicated by a blood test. I recommended the food sensitivity test.

He was more than willing to comply as no one had helped him thus far. We discussed dietary substitutions and he returned for his follow up three months later. He was thrilled. He had lost thirty pounds and he was so happy to be empowered to know what foods caused his pain and distress. He had avoided them strictly and adhered to the recommendations. All was well... Or so I thought. His wife was quite upset. She sat in the opposite chair with a very closed off energy, her arms crossed about her chest and a stern look on her face. I turned to her and said, "Aren't you happy that he is doing so well?"

"Oh yes!" She replied. "He is doing great, but since I have been cooking for him I have gained twenty pounds!"

I was confused. "How could cooking for him, the clean and healthy foods that I recommended while avoiding his trigger foods have caused her to gain weight? Was something else going on?" Then I realized that maybe there was a recurring theme to this weight loss I had witnessed in patients who had complied with the dietary recommendations. Maybe hers were different? And so I recommended that we test her, to which she was reluctant but agreed.

To my amazement her list of foods that she was sensitive too was almost completely opposite of his. I realized in that moment the power this food sensitivity program. She was willing to try to make meals separately for each of them and at her three month follow she had lost the extra twenty she had gained plus ten more pounds. "Holy Crap!" I thought! "This is huge!"

I had personally gained almost eighty pounds on synthetic hormones after my hysterectomy and when I went on bio-identical hormones and started exercising I had lost all but the last fifteen or twenty pounds. I thought to myself that I would do the test and see if this really worked. So I did... **and it did**! I am down to 130 pounds and follow my list very closely and feel wonderful. Years of stomach pain and IBS and struggling with my weight were gone. I have since used this strategy on thousands of patients and get consistent results as long as the patient understand, believes and adheres to the test and follows it. I have been giddy with the discovery until I went to my annual continuing education courses at the anti-aging conference and learned that many doctors all over the world are using the food sensitivity results for weight loss. I had patted myself on the back for discovering this and felt quite deflated in that I did not really discover anything at all.

We have created a whole program around food sensitivities and continue to get incredible results. "So how does this work?"

The inability to tolerate certain foods also known as sensitivity or intolerance, induces chronic activation of the immune system. Free radicals are produced and mediators of inflammation. This inflammation has been linked to countless chronic conditions, including: digestive disorders, migraines, obesity, chronic fatigue, attention deficit issues, aching joints, skin disorders, arthritis and many more.

This inflammation induces a cortisol response from the adrenal glands which ultimately leads to unwanted belly fat. (see section on hormones)

How does food sensitivity differ from classic food allergies?

True or immediate food allergies refer to foods that trigger the immune system to acutely produce massive amounts of the chemical histamine that leads to anaphylaxis, a potentially fata condition that may cause the throat and esophagus to swell, cutting off air from the lungs, or may simply cause hives, rashes, and other non-life-threatening reactions.

This type of reaction is called a hypersensitivity reaction, caused by the degranulation of mast cells or basophils that is mediated by Immunoglobulin E (IgE). This happens within in minutes. Then there is a delayed reaction that can take up to 3 days to appear. This is mediated by the part of the immune system called IgG.

Food allergies are divided into two major categories: immediate and delayed. Delayed can take up to 72 hours to appear. Some people get confused about food allergies versus sensitivities. When we talk of the delayed response we often refer to this as a "sensitivity" or "food intolerance".

Non-IgE-mediated food hypersensitivity (food intolerance) is more chronic, less acute, less obvious in its presentation, and often more difficult to diagnose than a food allergy. Symptoms of food intolerance vary greatly, and can be mistaken for the symptoms of a food allergy.

While true allergies are associated with fast-acting immunoglobulin IgE responses, it can be difficult to determine the offending food causing a food intolerance because the response generally takes place over a prolonged period of time. Thus the causative agent and the response are separated in time, and may not be obviously related. Food intolerance symptoms usually begin about half an hour after eating or drinking the food in question.

Food intolerance can present with symptoms affecting the skin, respiratory tract, gastrointestinal tract either individually or in combination. On the skin may include skin rashes, itching, hives, swelling and chronic eczema. Respiratory tract symptoms can include a stuffy nose, sinus infections, asthma, and cough among many. Gastrointestinal symptoms may include ulcers in the mouth, reflux or chest pain (heart burn), abdominal cramps, nausea, gas, bloating, intermittent diarrhea or constipation (irritable bowel symptoms-IBS) and vomiting or even prolonged gastritis, bleeding, hemorrhoids, ulcers and chronic gastrointestinal pain.

Other symptoms include headaches, joint and muscle pains and lead to more insidious disease from the inflammation like cancer, aging and cardiovascular disease (heart attacks and strokes).

So if you have any symptoms there are a couple things you can do to test to see if you have food sensitivities.

FIFTEEN/FIFTEEN Rule: One quick and dirty test you can do is to get a stop watch and monitor your pulse for one minute. If you eat something you are sensitive to your pulse will go up fifteen or more beats within fifteen minutes. The problem with this is that it is sensitive but not specific. You won't know what food triggered you. If you eat multiple foods it could be any one of them. You can experiment with different isolated foods to do this test. The problem is that it has to be a pretty severe sensitivity to trigger a response this quickly. Some of the milder triggers may take up to three days to trigger this response.

One other way you can try is elimination diet but this can be tricky because often when someone gives up one food they often eat more of something else they could be triggered by.

The other option and a much more reasonable option is just to have your blood tested. This is sensitive and specific and spot on every time.

How do you test for them?

This is measured as IgG, unlike IgE (immediate response/ allergy). This is a delayed response by the immune system. To verify if you have an IgG food intolerance a simple blood test can be done to identify 100 to 200 foods. The test examines the blood directly. A blood sample is taken, the lab technician identifies delayed onset allergies by observing how white blood cells and red blood cells react if they are exposed to selected foods. Red and white blood cell samples literally explode when allergens are introduced. What is also excellent around the allergy test is that the test will not be tied to detecting food intolerances; it may also identify reactions to artificial additives, antibiotics, environmental chemicals, and pharmacological ingredients.

The process measures the amount of response as well as if there is a response of your white blood cell antibodies (IgG) to protein substance (antigens) in the specific foods tested.

This is a sample food allergy test panel from Alletess, the company we use most often.

TEST	SCORE	CLASS		TEST	SCORE	CLASS	
ALMOND	0.179	0		LETTUCE	0.158	0	
APPLE	0.159	0		LOBSTER	0.170	0	
ASPARAGUS	0.175	0		MALT	0.157	0	
AVOCADO	0.157	0		MILK (COW'S)	0.310	2	**
BANANA	0.161	0		MUSHROOM	0.211	1	*
BARLEY	0.263	1	*	MUSTARD	0.168	0	
BASIL	0.170	0		NUTRA SWEET	0.157	0	
BAY LEAF	0.160	0		OAT	0.166	0	
BEAN (GREEN)	0.172	0		OLIVE (GREEN)	0.155	0	
BEAN (LIMA)	0.176	0		ONION	0.161	0	
BEAN (PINTO)	0.289	1	*	ORANGE	0.172	0	
BEEF	0.168	0		OREGANO	0.155	0	
BLUEBERRY	0.150	0		PEA	0.182	0	
BRAN	0.155	0		PEACH	0.148	0	
BROCCOLI	0.222	1	*	PEANUT	0.151	0	
CABBAGE	0.163	0		PEAR	0.139	0	
CANTALOUPE	0.190	0		PEPPER (BLACK)	0.151	0	
CARROT	0.172	0		PEPPER (CHILI)	0.153	0	
CASHEW	0.213	1	*	PEPPER (GREEN)	0.151	0	
CAULIFLOWER	0.206	1	*	PINEAPPLE	0.266	1	*
CELERY	0.149	0		PORK	0.127	0	
CHEESE (CHEDDAR)	0.144	0		POTATO (SWEET)	0.145	0	
CHEESE (COTTAGE)	0.141	0		POTATO (WHITE)	0.147	0	
CHEESE (SWISS)	0.146	0		RICE	0.137	0	
CHICKEN	0.155	0		RYE	0.206	1	*
CINNAMON	0.122	0		SAFFLOWER	0.149	0	
CLAM	0.139	0		SALMON	0.184	0	
COCOA	0.209	1	*	SCALLOP	0.146	0	
COCONUT	0.173	0		SESAME	0.139	0	
CODFISH	0.151	0		SHRIMP	0.159	0	
COFFEE	0.266	1	*	SOLE	0.190	0	
COLA	0.144	0		SOYBEAN	0.144	0	
CORN	0.141	0		SPINACH	0.143	0	
CRAB	0.231	1	*	SQUASH	0.145	0	
CUCUMBER	0.159	0		STRAWBERRY	0.142	0	
DILL	0.151	0		SUGAR (CANE)	0.134	0	
EGG WHITE	0.290	1	*	SUNFLOWER (SEED)	0.136	0	
EGG YOLK	0.193	0		SWORDFISH	0.147	0	
EGGPLANT	0.161	0		TEA (BLACK)	0.163	0	
GARLIC	0.141	0		TOMATO	0.156	0	
GINGER	0.256	1	*	TUNA	0.200	1	*
GLUTEN	0.319	2	**	TURKEY	0.151	0	
GRAPE	0.150	0		WALNUT (BLACK)	0.166	0	
GRAPEFRUIT	0.161	0		WATERMELON	0.162	0	
HADDOCK	0.147	0		WHEAT	0.310	2	**

You can see on this test that the foods in red have triggered an IgG reaction in this patient and it is rated 1, 2 or 3. The higher the number the more reactive the patient is to that food. 3 is the worst, or 3 stars or the higher the number the worse the reaction.

During your detox you avoid all foods in red and afterward in the rotation schedule you rotate foods with a 1 or 2 every 3-5 days and avoid 3's. The rationale for this is that it takes approximately 3 days to develop a new IgG antibody/antigen protein reaction, giving your body time to reset the inflammatory response.

How do I proceed with my new diet? How do I know if ingredients are present in prepackaged foods that I eat? This is a sample of an ingredient label. You must read all labels very carefully. Even things that you would not suspect like vitamins and supplements may contain foods that you may be sensitive to. You have to read all labels. I was watching a show on the Discovery channel where they were making sausage and they were putting gluten in it to make it look like more food. They call these fillers or thickeners. Even cosmetics may have foods that you are sensitive to. The ingredient list on a food label is the listing of each ingredient in descending order of predominance.

Detoxification Protocol Program

Finding out your food sensitivities is a wonderful gift! You now know the right fuel to put in your tank! You will never be the same again. Though you may be shocked and scared when you first see the list (this is normal, everyone reacts with a little shock and fear) you will now know what you need to know to begin changing your life, reducing inflammation and preventing disease due to inflammation. You are going to receive an abundance of wonderful and healthful benefits throughout the completion of your journey to wellness and improving your fertility.

The next step is the detoxification process and is outlined below. This is to cleanse the liver and digestive system, allowing your body to function at its fullest, get your hormones in balance and prepare your body for pregnancy.

We hope you will find this protocol easy to understand and follow.

Detoxification

The following diet plan is a sample plan. It is designed to avoid the BIG 8 food sensitivities. It should be followed as closely as possible. It is important that you avoid the foods that are on your food sensitivity list and take in the proteins, carbohydrates and fats as suggested. However, it can be altered and "moved around" to fit your needs. Be diligent, take control of your health and enjoy the benefits.

Once you have completed the detoxification program you will be able to start adding the foods that are 1's and 2's back into your diet on a rotation schedule.

Protein supplementation is a vital part of your detox program. During the detoxification phase, we ask that you use a specific type of protein for your program and lifestyle. The type of protein we now recommend to all of our patients is a high quality Brown Rice protein powder supplement. We recommend brown rice protein as it is easily digested and utilized. Brown rice protein does not cause any digestive or side effect issues like we see with Whey or Casein type protein supplements.

Sample Grocery List

(Remember: shop according to your food sensitivity list if you have it done)

- Filtered Water 3-6 gallons (See desired amount to drink from chart above)
- Fresh Limes &/or Lemons

- Organic Maple Syrup-Grade B
- Green Tea
- Protein Drink (Vegetable: Pea or Rice)
- Herbal Tea
- Turkey Breast (Organic if possible)
- Chicken Breast (Organic if possible)
- Fish-Tilapia, Salmon, Tuna, etc.
- Fresh fruit: Apples, pears, melons, berries, peaches, nectarines, kiwi, citrus. No bananas or mango.
- Almonds (Raw nuts and seeds are best)
- Cashews
- Sunflower seeds
- Pumpkin seeds
- Green vegetable
- Salad Greens
- Spinach
- Broccoli
- Cauliflower
- Squash
- Zucchini
- Carrots
- Onion
- Garlic
- Potato
- Sweet Potato
- Beans
- Peas
- French Vinaigrette Dressing or other suitable oil based dressing
- Olive oil
- Brown Rice
- Rice Crackers
- Organic Almond Butter or Cashew Butter
- Spices of any kind are acceptable for cooking
- Steel Cut Oats

21 DAY DETOXIFICATION PROTOCOL – Remember if you have had food sensitivity testing to substitute any foods that you are sensitive to.

PREPARATION PHASE 1 - SAMPLE MENU - *DAYS 1 TO 8*

Breakfast   Protein Shake 1 serving before breakfast

                  1 serving: Turkey or Chicken

                  OR 1 serving: Steel Cut Oatmeal or Gluten Free Rolled Oats (may use 1 packet of Stevia to sweeten) and 1 serving: Fresh Fruit (Stick with berries or pitted fruit)

Morning Snack   (Not mandatory) Nuts, animal protein and/or protein

                  supplement shake

Lunch   Fresh green or spinach salad with olive oil dressing (You can use this throughout the program)

                  Fish – broiled or baked

                  Steamed/ raw/grilled/baked vegetables

Afternoon Snack (Not mandatory) Nuts, animal protein and/or protein

                  supplement shake

Dinner   1 serving: Turkey or Chicken Breast or Fish – broiled steamed/ raw/grilled/baked vegetables, beans or peas,   salad

Nighttime Snack (Not mandatory) vegetable, almond butter or small

                  protein shake

FOODS TO EAT DURING THIS PHASE

- Drink plenty of fresh water (8-10 glasses), herbal teas, green tea
- Eat as much fresh cruciferous vegetables as you want (again watching your food sensitivities)
- Grain foods from rice, millet, quinoa, buckwheat, tapioca
- Fresh fruits, vegetables, beans, peas
- Fish, chicken, turkey *if* cold cuts-> (To truly detoxify Eat only organic /**no** additives/nitrates/nitrites/growth hormones/MSG/ preservatives
- Olive oil, flaxseed oil, coconut oil, all natural seasonings, sea salt

FOODS TO AVOID DURING THIS PHASE

- Any food that you know you are allergic/sensitive
- Dairy (milk, cheeses, yogurt, butter), eggs, margarine, shortening
- Foods prepared with Gluten-containing cereals like wheat, oats, rye, barley, those ingredients normally found in breads, pasta, etc.
- Tomatoes and tomato sauces, corn (GMO), peanuts
- Alcohol, caffeine (coffee, black tea, soda), sweeteners
- Soy products, beef, pork, conventional cold cuts (Oscar Mayer), bacon, hotdogs, canned meat, sausage, shellfish, meat substitutes, shellfish
- Fried food, dried fruit or fruit juices

DETOXIFICATION PHASE 2-SAMPLE MENU - *DAYS 8 TO 14* (No animal protein)

Note: This phase is important to remove animal protein from the diet for allowing the liver and system to reset. It can be a difficult time for fatigue and set-backs. But it is very important. We recommend that you do this every 3-6 months to detoxify the system.

Breakfast   Protein Shake 1 serving before breakfast

Steel Cut Oatmeal & Fruit or Gluten Free Rolled Oats

Morning Snack   Carrot sticks or celery & protein shake

Protein Shake   1 serving before lunch

Lunch   Salad with nuts, seeds, avocado/Olive Oil Dressing

Steamed/ raw/grilled/baked vegetables

Afternoon Snack   Fresh fruit or nuts & protein shake

Dinner   Protein Shake 1 serving before dinner Baked Potato or Baked Sweet Potato

Brown rice & Steamed/ raw/grilled/baked vegetables, beans, peas

Salad

Nighttime Snack   (Not mandatory) vegetable, almond butter or small

protein shake

FOODS TO EAT DURING THIS PHASE

- Drink plenty of fresh water (8-10 glasses), herbal teas, green tea
- Eat as much cruciferous vegetables as you wish (according to food sensitivities)
- Grain foods from rice, millet, quinoa, buckwheat, tapioca
- Fresh fruits, vegetables, beans, peas
- Olive oil, flaxseed oil, coconut oil, all natural seasonings, sea salt

FOODS TO AVOID DURING THIS PHASE

- _**ALL ANIMAL PRODUCTS**_-fish, turkey, chicken
- Any food that you know you are allergic
- Dairy (milk, cheeses, yogurt, butter), eggs, margarine, shortening
- Foods prepared with Gluten-containing cereals like wheat, oats, rye, barley, those ingredients normally found in breads, pasta, etc.
- Tomatoes and tomato sauces, corn, peanuts
- Alcohol, caffeine (coffee, black tea, soda), sweeteners
- Soy products, beef, pork, conventional cold cuts (Oscar Mayer), bacon, hotdogs, canned meat, sausage, shellfish, meat substitutes,
- Fried Food, dried fruit, fruit juice

******(NOTICE PROTEIN IS RE-INTRODUCED)*****

COMPLETION PHASE 3 - SAMPLE MENU-_DAYS 15 TO 17_

Breakfast	Protein Shake 1 serving before breakfast 1 serving: _**Turkey**_ or _**Chicken**_
	or
	1 serving: Steel Cut Oatmeal or Gluten Free rolled oats (may use 1 packet of Stevia to sweeten)
	and 1 serving: Fresh Fruit (Stick with berries or pitted fruit)
Morning Snack	(Not mandatory) Nuts, _**animal protein**_ or _**protein**_ supplement shake
Lunch	Green or spinach salad with _**chicken breast**_/ Olive Oil dressing
	Steamed/ raw/grilled/baked vegetables

Afternoon Snack   (Not mandatory) Nuts, *animal protein* or *protein* supplement shake

Protein Shake 1 serving before dinner

Dinner   1 serving: *Fish* or *Chicken breast* or *Turkey*

Brown rice & Steamed/ raw/grilled/baked vegetables or beans/peas

Green salad

Nighttime Snack   (Not mandatory) vegetable, almond butter or small protein shake

FOODS TO EAT DURING THIS PHASE

- Drink plenty of fresh water (8-10 glasses), herbal teas, green tea
- Eat as much cruciferous vegetables as you wish
- Grain foods from rice, millet, quinoa, buckwheat, tapioca
- Fresh fruits, vegetables, beans, peas
- Fish, chicken, turkey *if* cold cuts-> (Organic /**no** additives/nitrates/ nitrites/growth hormones/msg/preservatives
- USDA Certified organic is best or Farmer's Market Produce)
- Olive oil, flaxseed oil, coconut oil, all natural seasonings, sea salt

FOODS TO AVOID DURING THIS PHASE

- Any food that you know you are allergic
- Dairy (milk, cheeses, yogurt, butter), eggs, margarine, shortening
- Foods prepared with Gluten-containing cereals like wheat, oats, rye, barley, those ingredients normally found in breads, pasta, etc.

- Tomatoes and tomato sauces, corn, peanuts

- Alcohol, caffeine (coffee, black tea, soda), sweeteners

- Soy products, beef, pork, conventional cold cuts (Oscar Mayer), bacon, hotdogs, canned meat, sausage, shellfish, meat substitutes, shellfish

- Fried food, dried fruit or fruit juices

COMPLETION PHASE 4 - SAMPLE MENU-*DAYS 18 TO 21*

Breakfast   Protein shake 1 serving before breakfast

1 serving: Turkey or Chicken

OR

1 serving: Steel Cut Oatmeal Gluten Free rolled oats (may use 1 packet of Stevia to sweeten)

AND 1 serving: Fresh Fruit (Stick with berries or pitted fruit)

Morning Snack   (Not mandatory) Nuts, animal protein or protein supplement shake

Lunch   Fresh green/spinach salad with Olive Oil dressing

Steamed/ raw/grilled/baked vegetables

Fish – broiled or baked

Afternoon Snack   (Not mandatory) Nuts, animal protein or protein supplement shake

Dinner   1 serving: Turkey or Chicken Breast or Fish – broiled or baked

Steamed/ raw/grilled/baked vegetables, beans or peas,   salad

Nighttime Snack   (Not mandatory) vegetable, almond butter or small protein shake

FOODS TO EAT DURING THIS PHASE

- Drink plenty of fresh water (8-10 glasses), herbal teas, green tea
- Eat as much cruciferous vegetables as you wish
- Grain foods from rice, millet, quinoa, buckwheat, tapioca
- Fresh fruits, vegetables, beans, peas
- Fish, chicken, turkey
- Olive oil, flaxseed oil, coconut oil, all natural seasonings, sea salt

FOODS TO AVOID DURING THIS PHASE

- Any food that you know you are allergic
- Dairy (milk, cheeses, yogurt, butter), eggs, margarine, shortening
- Foods prepared with Gluten-containing cereals like wheat, oats, rye, barley, those ingredients normally found in breads, pasta, etc.
- Tomatoes and tomato sauces, corn, peanuts
- Alcohol, caffeine (coffee, black tea, soda), sweeteners
- Soy products, beef, pork, conventional cold cuts (Oscar Mayer), bacon, hotdogs, canned meat, sausage, shellfish, meat substitutes, shellfish
- Fried food, dried fruit or fruit juices

Congratulations, AGAIN!! Now that you have reached this point, you have accomplished some major victories in regaining your health and vitality. You have completed Phase 1 and 2. You may not realize it, but you have:

1. Eliminated common food sensitivities that may up-regulate the neuroendocrine-immune axis and lead to dis-ease;

2. Detoxified your system of accumulated toxins, heavy metals, metabolic debris, sludge & waste products;

3. Established a more functional environment for body systems:

4. Cleared pathways for better digestion, filtration, elimination, & receptor activity;

5. Prepared your body for better metabolism, weight management, & nutritional utilization.

Now you can begin to add (1's and 2's on your food sensitivity list) foods back into the diet one at a time. For the next month, keep a dietary journal (the 24 Hour Daily Nutrition Summary) of what you eat including meals, snacks and beverages. Use the food guide or go to www.calorieking.com or www.myfitnesspal.com to calculate your caloric intake. It is very important to "feed" your body good whole nutrient dense foods on a consistent basis (3-4x/day). Your body needs the appropriate caloric intake on a daily basis for your metabolism to work to optimum levels. You should now know that weight loss is not as simple as calories in-calories out. Many patients actually don't eat enough. By keeping this log, we can ensure you are getting what your body needs. Also record how you feel with the food that was eaten. Keep a record of your daily exercise routine.

Specific fertility supplementation is recommended (see chapter on supplements), it is for a specific reason. Be sure to follow the prescribed regimen. Additionally, a daily dose of protein supplement with repair enzymes and anti-inflammatories may be beneficial to your program and overall health. Drink one serving of vegetable protein drink just before breakfast, or as a mid-morning snack.

Remember, you now have a daily nutritional and exercise program and a care plan to provide your body with optimum nutrition, function, repair, recovery and wellness. This is part of your lifestyle now. Eat according to the plan laid out for you. Drink plenty of fresh water. Include nutritionally rich foods. Love and care for your body and it will respond the way you want. You have already come a long way and laid the foundation to the new YOU. Great job! Let's keep your progress going full steam ahead.

Pat yourself on your back! You did it!!!!

Now we need to focus on Exercise. You want to get healthy right?

Increase physical activity. Exercise! Yes, you will have to exercise if you want to get healthy and have lots of energy for that baby that is coming. No magic fairy dust here. It doesn't mean you have to go out and join a gym or buy expensive equipment. You must find something you can do without causing pain or injury.

Almost everybody can walk. You don't need a treadmill, if it is too cold outside. You can walk in your house. Everyone has a little space they can at least pace. There is no excuse. I love my exercise DVDs because I can do them in my living room in my underwear if I want. I like...*Turbo Jam, 10 minute solutions, exercise ball workout for dummies, the wave, and core rhythms...* Most of all, I love my Wii and the "*Just Dance*" programs. They are so much fun and easy to do. Just commit to 20 minutes 3-5 times a week and it will change your life.

If you only have a few minutes a day then strength training is going to give you your biggest bang for your buck! Muscle burns fat for you all day. If you are going to walk then interval training will maximize your workout. This just means walk as fast as you can for as long as you can without getting really winded (usually 2-5 minutes) and then walk at a brisk pace and alternate this activity.

You must be careful not to "over exercise" because if you push beyond your metabolic capabilities you become subject to a variety of ailments including tissue damage hormone imbalance immune system dysfunction or injury.

Exercise does not have to be vigorous or difficult but requires extra demand on your system which is not normally experienced. Many patients say "Well, I walk all day at work." As I said earlier, with extra demands (not normal experiences) your body will adapt to the new (good) stress and become conditioned, stronger and healthier. This means you should

Change your exercise routines regularly as well.

You must exercise correctly and learn how to do it without causing injury. You need to educate yourself and also know your goals. If you perform below your expectations on some days; it is ok. Your body has its own biorhythms and will fluctuate in energy and strength from one day to another.

The biggest thing is to do something you enjoy and just do it.

Exercise has been shown to improve immunity, reduce body fat, and improve mood states. It is a known fact; regular exercise improves glucose metabolism and insulin sensitivity one of the major issues in polycystic ovarian syndrome.

When our cells have adequate B vitamins, the brisk pace of methylation keeps homocysteine levels low. When we're low on those vitamins, homocysteine can build up quickly and slow or stop the production of SAMe and cause many problems with our health. High homocysteine is a major risk factor for heart attack and stroke. During pregnancy, it raises the risk of spina bifida and other birth defects. And many studies have implicated it in depression. Elevated homocysteine Increases inflammation and counters adequate attempts at the body to burn fat.

Omega-3 fatty acids (fish oil) studies have shown daily fish oil and moderate exercise are enough to influence weight loss even without other dietary changes. The Omega-3 fatty acids in oily fish can contribute to significant weight loss by increasing the elasticity of blood vessel walls and improving the flow of blood to muscles during exercise. Taking a 45-minute walk three times a week appears sufficient to produce the weight loss benefit.

Challenge equals change! You must constantly be changing and developing your body contour to burn fat and sculpt your image.

Here are some sample exercises for strength training. I recommend spending just 10-15 minutes a day for these reps.

My Favorite Exercises!

Aerobics: Wii-Just Dance 1 and 2, Wii-Zumba, Swimming, Walking, Dancing

Exercise Ball: Sit ups and crunches

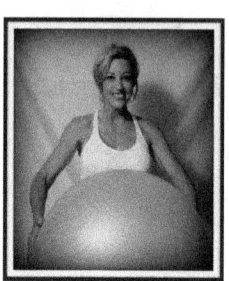 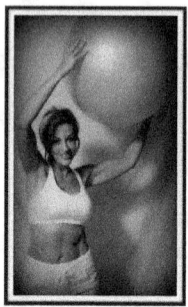 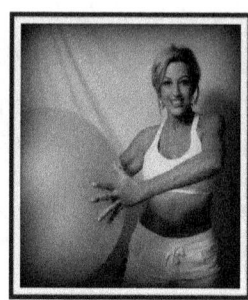

Exercise Ball: Round the world

Start with your exercise ball above your head, arms extended then rotate the ball clockwise for 5 reps then counterclockwise for 5 reps. A stay ball with sand in it really works your arms. Suck in your abs while you do this exercise for more ab work.

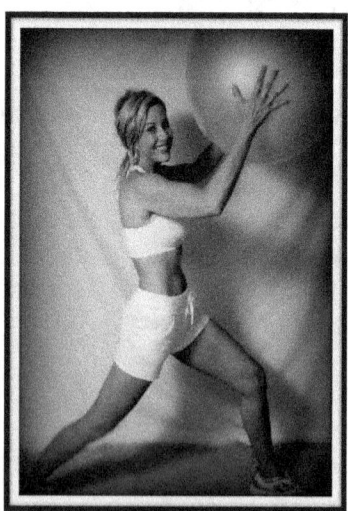

Lunges
Stand with ball in front of you and lunge forward then pull the ball into your extended knee and repeat 11 reps.

Push Ups

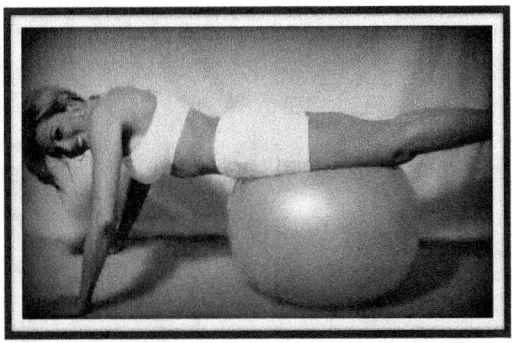

Kettle Bell: Round the world

Same things as with the ball but now with a heavier weight. Start
with 3lb. kettle bell. Never lift more than you can handle with
muscle fatigue.

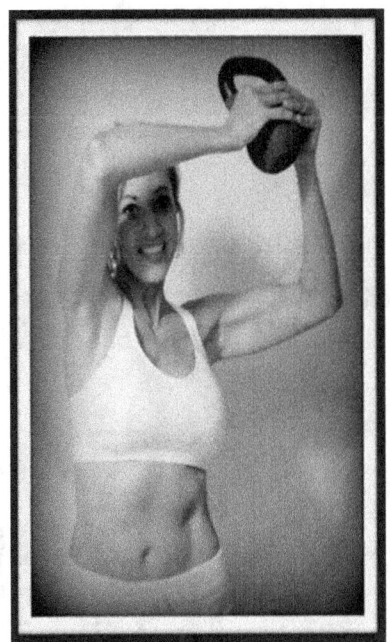
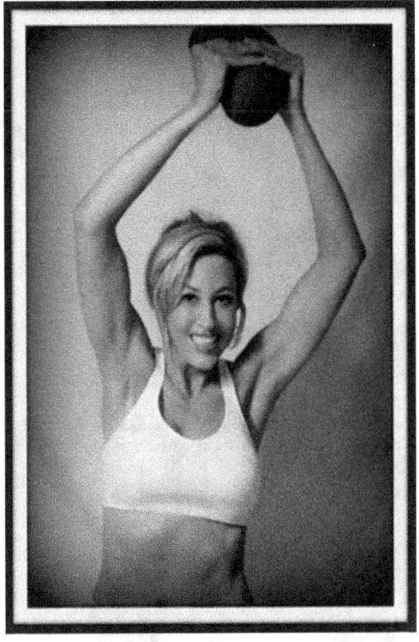

Ski Bumps

Hold kettle bell in front and bend knees, like you are going over little bumps while skiing

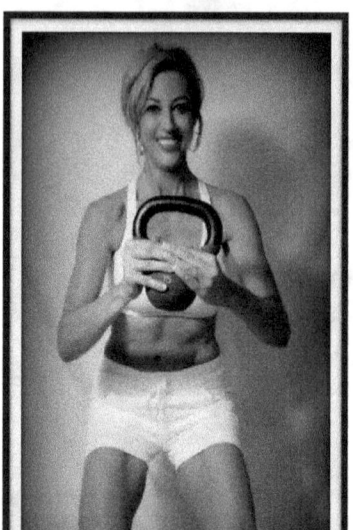

Hula-Hoop

Hold kettle bell in front and bend knees, like you are going over little bumps while skiing

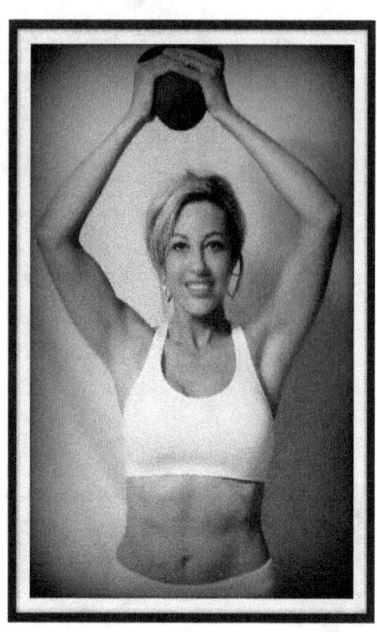

Throws

Kettle bell up over shoulder and drop down to opposite knee

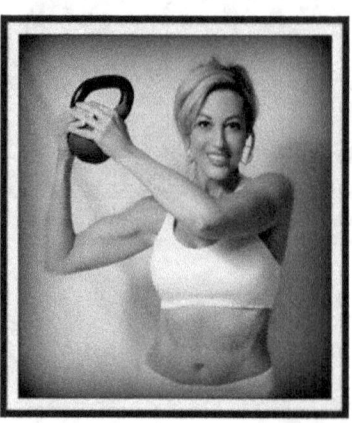

Drops

Kettle bell throws into the middle of the inner thighs and back out.

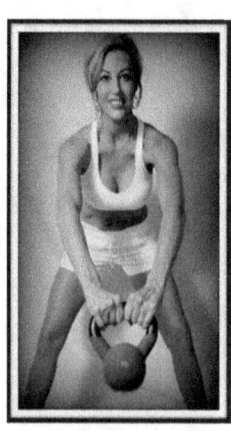

Band Froggies: Bend over with the band around your shoulders and feet. Keep your abs vertical with the floor and bend your knees.

Band Squats: Squat all the way to your knees, buttocks to ankles.

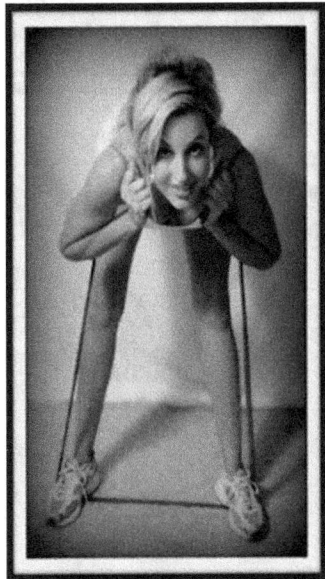

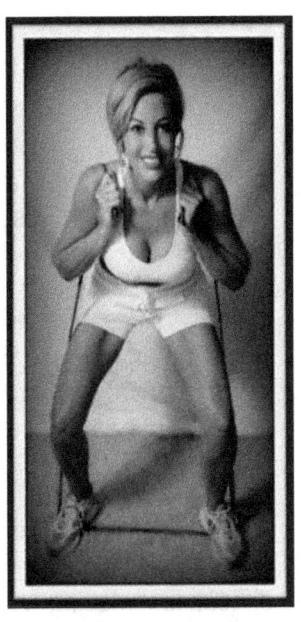

Band Lunges: Band stretched out, lunge deep bending back leg.

Band Side Bends: Use band to stretch side to side overhead.

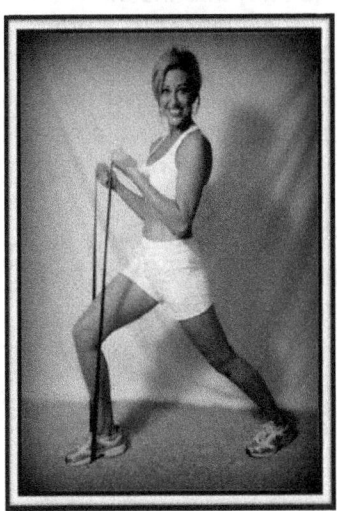

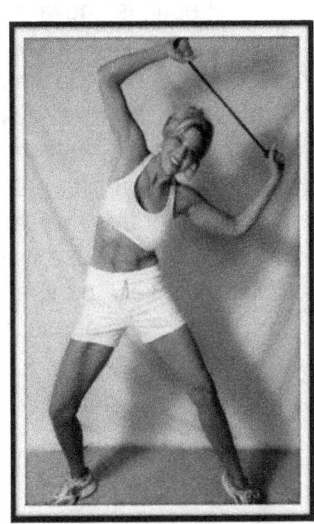

Band Donkey Kicks: Stretch band behind and kick out.

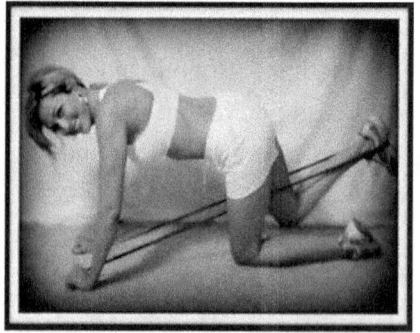

Sleep

To be healthy and balance your hormones sleep is an important topic. Researchers say that how much you sleep and how well you sleep may silently orchestrate a symphony of hormonal activity tied to your   appetite and overall hormone balance. According to the National Sleep Foundation, the average woman gets only six and a half hours of sleep per night. Chronic sleep deprivation can have a variety of effects on the metabolism and overall health.

You've heard it before. "Gotta get your beauty sleep". It's really true. If you don't get adequate sleep you will have a very difficult time losing weight and pregnant. The main reason is that when you don't get enough sleep a hormone called Ghrelin is released in excess. Ghrelin is a hormone that is known to stimulate appetite. Leptin is the yang of Ghrelin.

Leptin is known to decrease appetite and is abundant when sleep is adequate. Usually this is around 8-9 hours for the average adult. In 2006 at the American Thoracic Society International Conference, it was shown that women who slept 5 hours per night were 32% more likely to experience major weight gain (an increase of 33 pounds or more) and 15% more likely to become obese over the course of the 16-year study, compared to those who slept 7 hours a night. Those women who slept 6 hours per night were still 12% more likely to experience major weight gain and are 6% more likely to become obese, compared to women who slept 7 hours a night.

Just a few days of sleep restriction starts an abnormal cascade of hormone imbalances that increase hunger. Even if you eat less, you will still gain weight. Then, there is the impact of cortisol levels. When you don't get enough sleep, there is an increase in cortisol that also stimulates hunger, affects insulin and may therefore add to unwanted weight gain. It does this by decreasing the ability to process carbohydrates, manage stress, and maintain a proper balance of hormones. In just one sleep-restricted week, research study participants had a significant loss in their ability to process glucose and had an accompanying rise in insulin.

Your basal metabolic rate thermostat (calories you burn at rest) may be reset when you do not receive adequate sleep in a negative way. Also, those that don't rest well are tired and may not move around as much during the day to burn calories. Inadequate sleep can reduce levels of growth hormone that regulate the body's proportions of fat and muscle, so not only are you fat, but you'll be "lumpy".

As mentioned, sleep quality is important to assess as well. The hit show "The Biggest Loser" knows this, too. Since the show's seventh season, sleep studies have been added to the contestants' pre-show medical work-ups. Those with sleep apnea receive treatment. Doctors found that a majority of the contestants had sleep apnea, not surprising a neck measurement of 17 inches puts you at great risk, and often severe cases. In one season, every cast member had a positive sleep apnea diagnosis according to the National Sleep Foundation's website. This website has an interesting interview of Sean Algaier and how sleep apnea affected his life.

The Greek word "apnea" literally means "without breath." There are three types of apnea: obstructive, central, and mixed. Of the three, obstructive is the most common. Despite the difference in the root cause of each type in all three, people with untreated sleep apnea stop breathing   repeatedly during their sleep, sometimes hundreds of times during the night and often for a minute or longer.

Snoring is not normal. It runs the emotional gambit of cute to down right annoying to most. Marriages have ended over it. Some people think that it is okay to snore. It isn't. The sound of the snore is from a physical blockage of the airway or obstruction. Obstructive sleep apnea (OSA) is caused usually when the soft tissue in the rear of the throat collapses and closes during sleep. In central sleep apnea, the brain fails to signal the muscles to breathe. Mixed apnea, as the name implies, is a combination of the two. With each apnea event, the brain briefly arouses people with sleep apnea in order for them to resume breathing, but consequently sleep is extremely fragmented and of poor quality.

Sleep apnea is very common...

Risk factors include being male, overweight, and over the age of forty. It can affect anyone of any age, even kids. There seems to be an insurmountable lack of awareness by the public and healthcare professionals. The vast majority remain undiagnosed and therefore untreated, despite the fact that this serious disorder can have significant consequences like high blood pressure, congestive heart failure, Impotency, weight gain and headaches. Something else scary is that untreated sleep apnea could cause accidents at work or car wrecks from being sleep deprived and sleepy during the day. Fortunately, sleep apnea can be diagnosed and treated. Several treatment options exist. Sometimes, this is in the form of a mask called a CPAP that holds the airway open, surgery to remove extra tissues, and even sewing a tennis ball to your pajama back to prevent you from rolling onto your back.

Which came first, "The chicken or the egg?"... I sometimes wonder if obesity causes sleep apnea or if sleep apnea causes obesity. Either way it should always be addressed in any weight loss program.

Some people have a hard time going or staying asleep. You may need to address something called sleep hygiene. These are regular patterns that may assist you in going or falling asleep and include:

- Use the bedroom for sleep only. Don't use the bedroom as an office or for watching TV before bed. You want to reduce any stimulation when you are trying to wind down. One of the biggest mistakes people make in corrupting their sleep is to use their bedroom for activities other than sleep or sex.

- You should establish regular sleeping and waking times. Brain confusion can occur and shift workers have a really hard time with this issue. Have a bedtime routine like showering or washing your face, prayer, meditation, reading or deep breathing and relaxation.

- Avoid spicy food, caffeine, sugar and alcohol (Alcohol is initially sedating but causes CNS excitation later) at least 4 to 6 hours prior to going to sleep.

- Develop a regular exercise program. Exercise and good nutrition will help enhance sleeping patterns. However, avoid exercising 2 hours before sleeping, since this may stimulate your body and make sleeping more difficult.

- Block out distracting noises and lights. You are in your bedroom to sleep and not to be distracted by environmental interferences. Melatonin is a hormone that promotes sleep and is increased when the room is really dark.

- You may want to keep a sleep log that details your sleeping patterns, habits and improvements. This can be used and reviewed each time you find yourself with disrupted sleep patterns

- Do not smoke, especially if you are trying to get pregnant but this can interfere with sleep as well. Limit liquids after 8pm to avoid getting up to urinate. Drink a calming herbal tea such as chamomile or peppermint, unless urinating at night is an issue.

- Do not take your worries to bed - write them down and set aside a designated time to deal with them, and use comfortable bedding

- Sleep in a well-ventilated room that is neither too hot nor too cold. (A cooler room is better.) Avoid pets sleeping in the bed with you as they may interfere with a full night's sleep. Consider keeping them on the floor.

Stress

Emotional Stress is one of the biggest challenges that you will face in struggling with infertility. Focus on what you want! Don't give into the fear. If your life or health is not what you want it to be then you and only you can change it! You can't keep doing the same thing you've always done and expect it to change.

Healing, wellness and feeling fabulous is a journey. To be the fabulous you that you deserve to be you must make true change in your life. You must start your journey. You must embrace change.

Two things hold us back from making change: "Fear" and "Lack of Trust" To embrace change you may have to face your fears.

Fear can be protective, but what about when it keeps you from living the life you dream. What can you do about fear? How can you overcome it?

What are you afraid of? Do this exercise! It will change your life…

Write down on a piece of paper all the things you are afraid of. List them one by one. It can be a short list or long, but be honest. Then burn the list. Place it in a tin can with a glass of water near by and watch the paper slowly burn. Take a deep breath and let the ritual engulf you. Let it go. Let it all go! This is the first step. Then use the tips that follow to live your life in love and trust—NOT FEAR!

Face your fear to become stronger. SERIOUSLY? Or not? Don't take your fear so seriously. You might think to yourself that what you thought was a fear before wasn't that much to be afraid of at all. Everything is relative, and every triumph, problem, fear and experience becomes bigger or smaller depending to what you compare it to.

To gain a wider perspective of human experience and grow you really have to step up and face your fear. What if you don't have a baby? What would your life look like? Just be present with the thought. Don't try to push it under the rug.

2.   Take action and get busy. "Inaction breeds doubt and fear. Action breeds confidence and courage. If you want to conquer fear, do not sit home and think about it. Go out and get busy." Dale Carnegie.

Waiting and worrying about the fear helps nothing. Rally your troops. Get input from others. Make contact with the fear. Get in it's face. Start working on your health and learning as much as you can about how to change your health and your situation.

"Worry gives a small thing a big shadow." ...Swedish proverb

99% of the things we worry about happening, never happen and 99% of the things that happen, that we should have worried about, we never thought of.

3.   Focus on Love...When you hold others and make physical contact a hormone called oxytocin is released in the brain. This is the love hormone that helps moms to be affectionate and cuddle their babies. It is thought to be deficient in those with anxiety disorders and those with focus disorders or chronic pain, all physical manifestations of fear and lack of trust.

Here are ways to naturally boost your body's oxytocin production:

Hugs-Just embracing others, holding hands, or draping an arm around your significant other, child, or person you care for can produce an increase in oxytocin.

Make eye contact-When you interact with others oxytocin can be enhanced with mental embrace as well as physical contact.

Passion-Adults seeking an oxytocin surge should head for the bedroom. The hugging and touching during foreplay fires up the love chemical, and orgasm spikes the hormone level to two times the normal amount. This opens the door to a relaxed feeling and a greater opportunity to bond with your partner.

Get your hormones balanced-Interestingly, among premenopausal young women, oxytocin is naturally higher during ovulation because estrogen intensifies the love hormone. This may partially explain why women seem to be more prone to touch and other displays of affection during ovulation.

Daydream-Research out of the University of North Carolina at Chapel Hill discovered that happily married women quickly released a dose of oxytocin when asked to think about their husbands.

Get a pet- A loyal pet is there to make owners feel good and because the release of oxytocin is triggered by touch, petting a dog or cat you love can also increase oxytocin levels.

Get comfortable-Remember the smell of your mother's cookies, hearing kind words from someone you care about, telling someone how much you appreciate them, take a walk with a loved one—these are all ways to boost oxytocin.

You can also get oxytocin supplements if you have severe anxiety or fear issues.

4.   Fear is often based on false interpretation or miscommunication. As humans, it is our nature to look for patterns. The problem is just that we often find negative and not so helpful patterns in our lives based on just one or two experiences. Or by misjudging situations. Or through some silly miscommunication. Our brains make neuronal connections to past events. It is important not to judge past experience on future interactions. Every situation is different. We transfer a lot of fear and misgivings into future situations that we should really approach with a fresh perspective.

5.   Don't cling to your illusion of safety. The only thing permanent is change and there is no "comfort zone". One big reason why people don't face their fears is because they think they are safe where they are right now. But the truth is safety is only a sense, like fear, it is not real only perceived. There is no safety out there really. It is all uncertain and unknown.

Life happens, you may lose your job, your loved one, have to move, lose your home or suffer unknown tragedy. You may get laid off. You will eventually die. Who knows what will happen?
This perception of safety is not always a bad thing. It's protective. But there is also not that much point in clinging to an illusion of safety.

So you need to find balance where you don't obsessed by the uncertainty but also recognize that it is there and live accordingly.

As you stop clinging to your safety life also becomes a whole lot more exciting and interesting. You are no longer as confined by an illusion and realize that you set your limits for what you can do and to a large extent create your own freedom in the world. You are no longer building walls to keep yourself safe as those walls wouldn't protect you anyway.

6.   **Be curious-**"Curiosity will conquer fear even more than bravery will." James Stephens

When you are stuck in fear you are closed up. You tend to create division in your world and mind. You create barriers between you and other things/people.

How do you become more curious? One way is to remember how life has become more fun in the past thanks to your curiosity and to remember all the cool things it helped to discover and experience. And then to work at it. Curiosity is a habit. The more curious you are the more curious you become. And over time it becomes more of a natural part of you.

7.   **Trust-** the antidote to fear. Most of our fears are based on how others perceive us. The ego wants to divide your world. It wants to create barriers, separation and loves to play the comparison game. The game where people are different compare to you, the game where you are better than someone and worse than someone else. All of that creates fear. Doing the opposite removes fear.

But one thought you may want to try for a day is that everyone you meet is your friend. To take this one step further assume that every one you meet has something to teach you.

There is often an underlying frame of mind in interactions. Either it asks us how we are different to this person. Or how we are the same as this person. This creates warmth, an openness and curiosity within. There is no place to focus on fear or judgment anymore.

This is of course not easy, especially if you have held the first frame of mind for many years. But you can get insight into this by doing the rest of the things above. As you face your fears the barriers and separation you have built in your mind decreases. You come closer and feel more of a connection to other people.

With action, curiousness and understanding we come closer to each other. We gain a greater understanding of ourselves and others. And so it becomes easier to see them in you. And you in them.

Make your change. Don't hold on to your lack of fertility and your fear. Start the journey to a new you today! A fabulous YOU that will make a fabulous mom!

More about Oxytocin...

Oxytocin, is a peptide that functions as both a hormone and neurotransmitter, has broad influences on social and emotional processing throughout the brain and body. It has many implications with both weight loss and wellness. Oxytocin's role in reproductive functions is well known. In 1906, the English researcher Sir Henry Dale discovered a substance in the pituitary gland that could speed up the birthing process. He named it oxytocin from the Greek words for quick and child labor. Later, he found that it also promoted the expulsion of breast milk.

Now it appears that oxytocin plays a much larger physiological role than previously recognized, since under many circumstances, it has the ability to produce the effects that we associate with the state of calm and emotional wellbeing or connectedness.

Oxytocin is thought to be the yang of cortisol the stress hormone. Everyone needs oxytocin. Everyone's body was designed to release Oxytocin. Some of us have experienced stress and trauma to the point that our body's natural ability to create oxytocin is depleted. Nearly everyone experiences stress to a degree.

Love is the feeling and experience that ties us together. When we experience too much stress and anxiety in our lives, it breaks down vital relationships and leaves us feeling lonely and isolated. Adults who are under constant stress and anxiety experience more bouts of depression, dissatisfaction in life and increased health challenges.

In humans, oxytocin is released during hugging and pleasant physical touch. It plays a part in the human sexual response cycle. It appears to change the brain signals related to social recognition via facial expressions, perhaps by changing the firing of the amygdala, the part of the brain that plays a primary role in the processing of Important emotional stimuli. In this way, oxytocin in the brain may be a potent mediator of human social behavior.

In 1998 a study by Kovac was done that showed that Oxytocin reduced food cravings and sugar cravings, calms the mood and produces satiety sensations through counteracting stress.

As stated previously here are a few natural ways to increase your oxytocin:

- Share a warm hug or a kiss
- Cuddle
- Make love
- Sing
- Get or give a massage
- Hold a baby, a dog or cat
- Perform a generous act
- Pray or meditate
- Show support

Oxytocin plays a vital role in promoting factors that enhance well-being. Oxytocin plays a critical role at enhancing factors within the individual which promote well-being. Oxytocin induces increase in level of trust and reduction of fear through modulating the response of amygdala and other central structures to stress and fear. Oxytocin increases approach and pro-social behavior and enhances social interactions, as evidenced by human and animal studies. Oxytocin reduces subjective sense of anxiety, increases overall calm and is implicated in non-verbal intelligence.

The calm loving thoughts that you have will make a warm and oxytocin rich environment for your future baby.

Chapter Four

Getting pregnant naturally...

So you know about diet and balancing your hormones and getting healthy. Now let's get into the meat of how to prepare your body naturally to get pregnant.

It's no wonder this seems confusing and daunting. I am a doctor and I really had no clue how my own body really worked or how to fix it. Sure, I took biology and physiology, but no one ever told me what I really needed to know about hormones and the impact they have on the human body.

One day a patient came to my clinic, dressed professionally and quite eloquent with her words.

"Do you prescribe bio-identical hormones?" She asked

"Bio what?" I asked.

"You know," she paused "natural hormone therapy... like Suzanne Somers uses".

I had no idea what she was talking about, so I looked at her more intently, leaned in, and said, "Tell me more."

She proceeded to tell me about natural hormone therapy and all the benefits of it. I was astounded. My jaw dropped as she told about a world out there that was completely foreign to me. I thought hormone replacement therapy was bad, very bad. I thought it was only to be used for the woman who was soaking in sweat constantly or homicidal/suicidal.

I had received so much faulty information in medical school from pharmaceutical companies. They continue to feed us faulty information. Until that point, I believed a woman didn't need progesterone if she didn't have a uterus. I was taught there was only one way to take hormone replacement therapy and only a couple of different options or doses.

I told my patient I knew nothing about what she was talking about, and I promised her I would find out. I try to keep an open mind about alternative therapies. Many physicians don't bother with alternative therapies because there is already so much to learn and know. Why add more? These physicians ask, "If there is no evidence based research behind it (or at least that's what big pharmaceutical companies would have us believe), isn't it better to prescribe a pill?" Some doctors cattle forty or more patients through their halls a day. That doesn't leave much time to look into alternative therapies. I feel very differently about this and for this reason I vowed to look into "bio-identical hormone therapy".

I did a Google search on Suzanne Summers and soon had unlocked a door to a world I never knew existed. That was eight years ago. So, what was the outcome?

I started on bio-identical hormone therapy (and I prescribed it for that patient, too). I lost over sixty pounds and escaped night sweats and hot flashes! My mood was stable for once and I was sleeping again. I put testosterone in the prescription and actually got a libido back. I felt better than I had felt since those nasty periods started when I was a teenager.

I learned that my hysterectomy was probably not necessary. The abnormal pap, fibroids, and endometriosis found at the time of my surgery were all a product of my massive hormone imbalances. I learned my heavy periods were from the excess estrogen I was storing, when I unknowingly put on an extra ten pounds in college. From this and more, I have learned patients do not have to suffer and have unnecessary procedures, surgeries and rely on big pharmaceutical companies' answer to these issues.

So my journey began. I thank that woman every day for intriguing me with something new. I didn't know it that day, but I had embarked on a journey. Looking back, this time was the beginning of my true journey to wellness.

Over the past eight years, I have seen patients lose hundreds of pounds. People have transformed before my very eyes. Marriages have been healed from the ravages of hormonally imbalanced women AND men. I have been given a gift to be able to help people through this journey. I have sought out every aspect of metabolic realignment I could and this is the simplest presentation I have come up with.

To help you assess the severity of your hormone imbalance addressing the following list of symptoms or issues may help you monitor and keep track of your hormone balance. I have patient's check the box if they are having symptoms and then record Mild, Moderate, or severe after the response.

[] PMS (premenstrual syndrome) issues... cramps, nausea, breast tenderness, headaches, and/or irritability 1-2 weeks before my period

[] Difficulty falling asleep or staying asleep

[] Fatigue or loss of energy especially in the afternoon

[] Frequent bouts of irritability and depression

[] Frequent anxious feelings, anxiety attacks, or heart palpitations

[] Achy or stiff joints, especially in the morning

[] Gaining weight, especially around the middle

[] Losing weight is more difficult than in the past

[] Pain with intercourse

[] Inability to have orgasm, decreased sensitivity, or decreased sex drive

[] Vaginal dryness

[] Crave sweets, carbohydrates or alcohol.

[] Hair or skin that is dry, fragile, or thinning

[] Losing inches of height, diagnosed with osteoporosis, suffered from broken or fractured bones.

[] Recurrent yeast or urinary tract infections.

[] Irregular menstrual periods.

[] Hot flashes or night sweats.

[] Missing the outer third of your eyebrows

[] Frequent headaches or migraines

[] Fluid retention (rings fit tight or shoe size increased)

[] History of cysts on ovaries

[] Male distribution hair growth (facial hair, male pattern balding)

[] Problems with acne or rosacea

[] Heart racing or irregular heart beats felt

[] Hot or cold intolerance

[] Constipation or diarrhea

[] Frequent bouts of abdominal bloating or gas

[] Skin rashes or new onset allergies

In our program we use bio-identical hormones to correct the imbalances. For fertility issues we use bio-identical progesterone. Bio-identical progesterone hormone is manufactured in the lab to have the same molecular structure as the hormones made by your own body. By contrast, synthetic hormones are intentionally different. Drug companies can't patent a bio-identical structure, so they invent synthetic hormones that are patentable.

It's so unbelievable to me that bio-identical hormones have been around for years, although most doctors have never heard of them. Big pharmaceutical companies who have expensive patent-ed synthetic hormones would like to make sure they never do.

Most ovulation issues can be corrected by using bio-identical progesterone and for the simplicity of restoring ovulation and regular menstrual cycles we don't have to do extensive hormone testing, but if you want to truly know all the areas that may be in deficiency it can be a great way to do a more thorough evaluation.

Not every person needs hormone therapy. But in most cases of infertility, progesterone is deficient. That's why our simple program can be done without expensive lab testing and can be just as effective.

Many medical studies suggest that bio-identical hormones are safer than synthetic versions. It is often possible to rebalance hormones without the use of hormonal supplementation by using nutritional supplements, gentle endocrine support, and dietary and lifestyle changes.

Just a little about estrogen, although progesterone is at the root or lack there of, at the root of your ovulation issues and fertility issues. Not all estrogens are alike.....

Estrogen often gets a "bad rap" because of synthetic versions. Premenopausal women produce three biologically active estrogens, estrone (E1), estradiol (E2), and estriol (E3). Estradiol is the most abundant estrogen produced and both estrone and estradiol are potent estrogens. Estriol is considered a weak estrogen. Although little scientific data supports the claim, it has been postulated that estrone is a "bad" estrogen and may be the cause of estrogen's cancer-causing properties, while estriol is a "good" estrogen and may protect against cancer. Estradiol is probably neutral. Estrone can cause abnormal weight gain and interfere with getting pregnant.

Oral (taken by mouth) estrogens or progesterone, not given by systemic routes (patch, skin cream, vaginal cream, under the tongue), may be excessively converted into estrone with potential negative effects for the patient. Oral hormones, because they are metabolized by the liver, likely exert different effects than systemic estrogens which are not metabolized by the liver

Over 13 million women were on some form of synthetic HRT before the initial studies were published. When the studies came out millions quit "cold turkey". I can only imagine all those women and their symptoms returning. Many stayed on synthetic HRT, but live in fear of the consequences and hormone replacement therapy side effects. Many of those women were unnecessarily placed on antidepressants as pharmaceutical companies and doctors gained alliance to position those drugs as substitute products for lack of hormone balance. Most of these women were not depressed and now have been exposed to a new set of potential side effects.

The majority of studies published to date have concerned synthetic HRT. Both of these forms are usually take in pill form or orally. Studies have shown levels of CRP (c-reactive protein) are increased with intake of oral estrogen. CRP is a pro-inflammatory blood protein associated with increased risk of heart attack and stroke. Very few have involved or reported anything about bio-identical hormone replacement therapy. Oral estrogens are converted into estrone with potential negative effects; not estrogens given by transdermal or through the skin routes (patch, skin cream, vaginal cream, under the tongue).

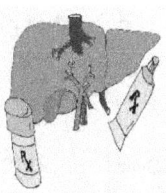

Why Creams and gels?

Oral hormones, with a focus on estrogen, are metabolized by the liver. This is known as first pass metabolism. When this happens a normal process occurs that creates "inflammatory proteins". These proteins can cause many different types of inflammation in the body. Of most concern are the blood vessels with a risk of a heart attack or a stroke.

When a route through the skin is chosen, this first pass metabolism by the liver is bypassed and goes straight to the tissues that need it. This is why we choose creams and gels.

Progesterone is usually the hormone that is deficient with infertility and this deficiency is at the root of many female menstrual cycle irregularities, pain, PCOS, endometriosis, and you bigger yet, you need progesterone to carry a pregnancy to term.

When you take progesterone in a pill form, most of it goes directly to the liver, where up to 80 percent of it may be dumped, but not before creating a variety of byproducts (metabolites). Thus, it's necessary to take 100 mg of progesterone in pill form to get 20 mg into your cells. If your liver happens to be working less efficiently on a given day, and excretes less of the progesterone, it's easy to experience overdose side effects; such as, sleepiness and bloating.

What they really need to do is use progesterone cream, which is a much more efficient delivery method. If you put 20 mg on your skin, virtually all of that will be in your bloodstream within a matter of minutes.

Progesterone and pregnancy: a vital connection

Progesterone is a natural female hormone. Called "the pregnancy hormone," it is essential before and during pregnancy. And after pregnancy to prevent "post partum depression".

Progesterone supplementation is often necessary during Assisted Reproductive Technology (ART) procedures, such as in-vitro fertilization (IVF) because the medications you may use during these procedures can suppress your body's ability to produce progesterone. Certain procedures can even, inadvertently, remove progesterone-producing cells from your ovaries. The problem with this is that they usually use synthetic versions of progesterone which can actually cause miscarriages and set you up for ovarian cancer and ovarian issues later in life.

Sometimes there are other reasons to use progesterone supplementation, such as little or no progesterone production from the ovaries or poorly developed follicles that do not secrete enough progesterone to develop the uterine lining. The bottom line is this

— all women who wish to become pregnant need progesterone to help the uterus prepare for and maintain a fertilized egg.

Before pregnancy – progesterone helps balance mood, weight and sleep. It prepares the uterus for implantation. Progesterone prepares the uterus for pregnancy. After ovulation occurs, the ovaries start to produce progesterone needed by the uterus. Progesterone causes the uterine lining or endometrium to thicken. This helps prepare a supportive environment in your uterus for a fertilized egg.

During pregnancy – Progesterone (from the root word, Pro-gestation or pro-pregnancy) keeps the system in alignment for maintaining the pregnancy. Progesterone helps nurture the fetus. A supply of progesterone to the endometrium continues to be important during pregnancy. Following a successful implantation, progesterone helps maintain a supportive environment for the developing fetus. After 8 to 10 weeks of pregnancy, the placenta takes over progesterone production from the ovaries and substantially increases progesterone production

Forms of progesterone

Several types of progesterone are available, including topical creams (very effective and easy to use) and vaginal products that deliver progesterone directly to the uterus. The different forms include the following:

Progesterone cream

- Used once a day for progesterone supplementation
- Is cycled to use 15 mg days 1-11 of menstrual cycle and then 25-30 mg during ovulation week and then back to 15 mg days 21-28.
- Over a decade of experience and over 40 million doses prescribed
- In studies where patient preference was measured, a majority of women preferred the cream for comfort and convenience over other progesterone formulations
- Progesterone is an important part of infertility treatment because it

- Most women prefer a progesterone formulation that is easy, convenient, and comfortable.

Saliva Testing? What's that all about???

Saliva testing has become the most specific way to assess the hormone levels in your tissues. Blood tests show only fluctuating levels from minute to minute. A full assessment of multiple hormones can be tested. It is easy to do. Although some insurance does not pay for it; these tests can be more affordable than blood tests in some cases.

Saliva testing is a convenient, inexpensive, and above all, accurate means of testing steroid hormones. Scientific studies have shown a strong correlation between steroid hormone levels in saliva and the amount of hormone in the blood that is active or "bioavailable." Saliva is an ideal diagnostic medium to measure the bioavailable levels of steroid hormones active in the tissue. It is this fraction of total hormone that is free to enter the target tissues in the brain, uterus, skin, and breasts.

Saliva testing can be done anywhere, anytime. Testing that relies on blood drawn in the doctor's office makes it harder to obtain samples at specific times (such as in the early morning) or multiple times during the day. In addition, hormones in saliva are exceptionally stable and can be stored at room temperature for up to a week without affecting the accuracy of the result. This offers maximum flexibility in sample collection and shipment. Several of the steroid hormones can be tested in the saliva including, estradiol, estrone, estriol, progesterone, testosterone, DHEA-S, and cortisol.

When a woman experiences prolonged stress, pregnenolone (that comes from the precursor cholesterol), a hormone essential for both coping with stress and producing female hormones, is diverted from the normal hormone pathway. As a result, the production of female hormones is compromised. This condition can cause a multitude of symptoms including irritability,

Each person is different and the whole person and hormonal chemical make-up and balance are unique. The doctor must take into account all the different complexities of an individual's hormone make-up and balance and work with what the person has in their environment to maximize the hormonal balance.

The hormonal health of any woman depends upon the delicate dance of progesterone and estrogen. Estrogen is meant to be the predominant hormone in the first half of the menstrual cycle and progesterone the predominant one in the second half. However, for most women in the industrialized world this is not the case.

There are many causes of hormone imbalance, but at the base of the problem is something called Estrogen Dominance - which means there is too much estrogen and not enough progesterone present in the body. There are many *symptoms* that result from having low progesterone levels.

What follows is a look at some of the common ways in which medicine and industry have tampered with the natural balance of our hormones. Women have used these products blindly at the cost of our hormonal balance, overall health, and longevity. Some of these may be obvious to you, while some may come as a surprise. Either way the hormonal imbalances that result should not be taken lightly. They contribute to the rise in cancers, especially breast and ovarian cancers, heart disease, depression, PMS and more.

The common causes of hormonal imbalance and estrogen dominance:

- Artificial hormone replacement therapy (The Pill and Prempro)
- Environmental poisons
- Non organic and estrogen pumped animal products
- Stress

- Cosmetics (chemicals in them that mimic estrogen in the Progestin's and progestogens (artificial/synthetic progesterone) are highly toxic to the body, resulting in some of these known side effects:

- miscarriages

- migraines

- heart disease

- high blood pressure

- cancer

- depression

and, of course ... lowers natural progesterone, the true biologic hormone levels.

These are some of the common ways that medicine has tampered with the natural balance of hormones, here are some the ways that industry has tampered with the same delicate hormonal balance.

Chemicals such as pesticides mimic the hormone estrogen. Fifty-one chemicals have now been identified as hormone disruptors. Approximately 2 billion tons of pesticides are used the annually the world over. In undeveloped countries, the use of pesticides is still largely unchecked and ... guess what? That is where we get a lot of our food supplies. It's plain to see why this is wreaking havoc on our bodies. It is this fact that has led many people to switch to an organic diet.

Other chemicals that cause the same challenges are DDT, dioxin and PCB's (polychlorinated biphenyls.) Dioxin is the by-product of the manufacture of chemicals using chlorine and includes:

- disinfectants

- dry cleaning fluids

- pesticides

- drugs

- plastics – polystyrene and cling wrap in particular

PCB's are used in: Lubricants

- plastics
- paints
- varnishes
- inks

Commonly called petrochemicals, they contain high levels of xeno-estrogens. Xeno-estrogens basically mean they mimic estrogen in your body. They fill up all the estrogen receptor sites in your body; even the good estrogen can't get through to perform its role properly. This results in hormone imbalance. This is why many people have moved over to household cleaning products that don't contain these chemicals and are environment friendly. Non-organic animals that are slaughtered for our food chain are fed estrogenic steroids to fatten them up. These estrogens go straight into our blood stream causing a further rise in estrogen levels. Another study linked the increase of our current disease rates to eating a diet high in the fat and meat from these estrogen-fed animals. Again, it is this fact that has led many people to switch to an organic diet. Cosmetics may come as a surprise to you, but many cosmetics are made with petro-chemicals, yes like you put in your car. It's not surprising then to re-alize that these 'moisturizers' are actually drying out your skin - actu-ally causing more wrinkles!

Even more importantly they are further putting your hormones out of balance. Just to list a few aqueous cream, petroleum jelly, mineral oil, liquid paraffin, talc powders, parabens, and other estro-genic antioxidants

Again, this is why many people have moved over to moisturizers that don't contain these chemicals and are environment friendly. As if all of the above where not enough, stress also plays a big part in reduc-ing our levels of progesterone which results in ... too much estrogen.

Here's how: Progesterone is the "mother of all hormones." It is the precursor and essential raw material out of which the body creat-ed ALL THE OTHER HORMONES. As the precursor to all the other hormones in the body, the adrenal glands and adrenal hormones are no exception. If you encounter a mildly stressful situation your body draws on its progesterone to produce the hormones (adrenal cortico-steroids) to counteract it. These are the hormones that protect against stress. BUT, if your body is in a constant or permanent state of stress it can't provide enough progesterone to be converted into anti-stress hormones and the result is adrenal exhaustion and no left over progesterone for other normal body functions. You can change your life! You can restore balance. You can combat aging and ill health effects starting today.

Here's how to use your progesterone cream in our Easy to use Fertility system:

Ovulation occurs at the point in a woman's menstrual cycle when a mature egg is released from the ovary and travels down the fallopian tube, ready to be fertilized if it meets a sperm cell. Since ovulation is the time when it is possible to get pregnant, it can be very useful to know how to calculate it.

A woman's most fertile days to conceive are influenced by her menstrual cycle and the lifespan of human eggs and sperm. The menstrual cycle has 3 phases: follicular, ovulatory and luteal phases.

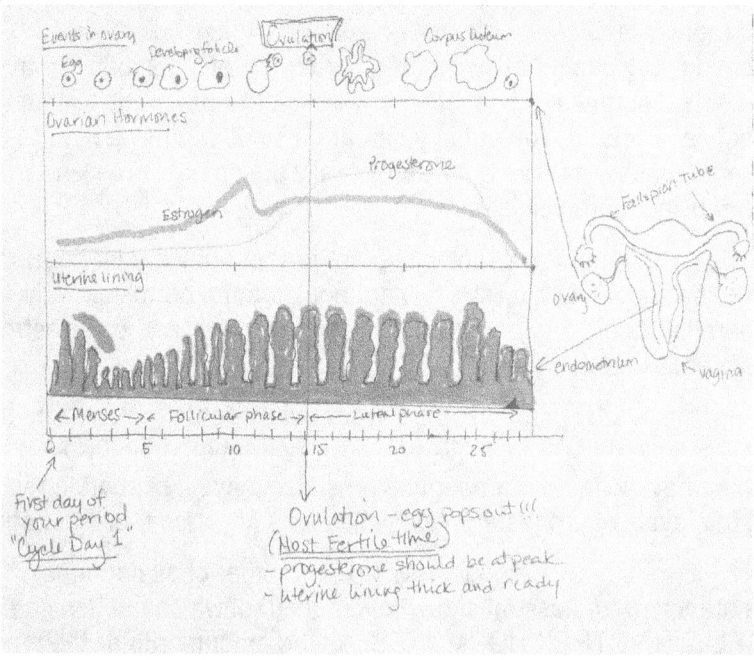

During the follicular phase, 15 to 20 eggs begin to mature in each ovary. Each egg is encased within a follicle, and the follicles produce the hormone estrogen. As the estrogen levels in a woman's body rise, the estrogen threshold is eventually reached which causes a surge in luteinizing hormone (LH). The LH surge causes ovulation, when the most mature egg is released into one of the Fallopian tubes.

After ovulation, the follicle that released the egg collapses on itself and begins producing the hormone progesterone, starting the luteal phase. The collapsed follicle is known as the corpus luteum and has a finite lifespan of 12 to 16 days if the egg is not fertilized. The progesterone prevents sperm from fertilizing any additional eggs during that cycle. To conceive, sperm must reach the mature egg before it dies. A typical egg can live 12 to 24 hours after ovulation, while sperm can survive up to 5 days in a hospitable vaginal environment. Your fertile days are the 5 days preceding ovulation and up to 2 days after ovulation. Methods to determine fertile cycle days use average cycle length, fertility signs, and hormone changes during the menstrual cycle.

Summary: Day 14 is the day you ovulate. We use the progesterone cream in a cycled fashion to enhance ovulation. If you see on the chart that estrogen peaks and if you already have too much estrogen from imbalance we use progesterone to promote ovulation to occur.

How to use the Endocreme: Start charting the length of your menstrual cycle. Keeping track of your cycle's duration can allow you to see the typical length of your follicular and luteal phases and help you pinpoint ovulation in the future to ensure regular cycles.

1. Use a calendar or spreadsheet to record the date of the first day of your period. This is day 1 of your menstrual cycle.

2. Continue to number each day of your cycle.

3. Start over with day 1 of the next cycle once your period begins again.

4. Chart for a minimum of 3 to 4 months. The more cycles you chart, the more reliable your assessment of your fertile days will be, but you need to track a minimum number of cycles to determine if your menstrual cycle is regular or irregular and how well the progesterone is working

The great news is your periods will be lighter and may only last 3 days. Yay!!! This is completely normal and the first month or two you may not have a period at all so don't be alarmed your body is just resetting itself.

Day 1-11 of menstrual cycle use ¼ dropper of the All Natural progesterone cream (we use Endocreme900 ™ -this formulation is medical grade but does not require a prescription) for our patients which is a topical progesterone. One dropper full is about 30 mg of Natural progesterone, so ¼ dropper is about 7.5 mg of progesterone.

Day 12-21 of menstrual cycle use full dropper about 30 mg and this will calm the estrogen effect and promote ovulation and support implantation.

Day 22-28 of menstrual cycle resume the ¼ dropper and then start the process all over again.

If your periods are irregular you simply need to just start counting days and within a month or two you should have regular light periods and ovulating regularly. Day 1 is the first day you start bleeding. Don't worry if it is irregular the first few months. Just follow the schedule. If you haven't had a period in several months then just start using the cream anytime and consider it day 1.

If you miss a day, don't stress just resume the next day or you can double the dose of the phase you are in for that day.

If your periods are heavy then adjust the dose down by just a few drops. If you have any side effects of headache or mood changes adjust the dose down as well.

You will want to get a calendar and plot out your days. Or you can use website menstrual trackers.

I recommend the following:

www.babymed.com

www.fertilityfriend.com

www.ovulation-calender.com

Other tracking that you may want to do that will help you identify your ovulation are as follows.

The easiest way, but may be a little more expensive as the methods that follow are free but take a little work on your part, is get an ovulation kit.

Get an Ovulation Kit

Use an ovulation predictor kit. Go by the manufactures directions. How do they work? Ovulation predictor kits typically provide test strips that indicate whether you have luteinizing hormone (LH) in your urine. The LH surge causes ovulation, is stimulated by progesterone, so the predictor kit will show once you have ovulated. This method will not show you your fertile days preceding ovulation.

•Open the kit and read the enclosed directions.

•Collect a urine sample and insert the test strip in the sample, or urinate on the test strip. Follow the method indicated for your specific kit.

•Wait to see if the strip indicates the presence of LH. Rising levels of LH indicate that egg will be released shortly.

Record your cervical mucus

Track changes in your cervical fluid. Cervical fluid changes in amount, look, consistency, and feel throughout the menstrual cycle in response to the hormones produced during different cycle phases.

•Check for cervical fluid each day. You can get a sample of the secretions by wiping front to back with a piece of toilet paper or by inserting a clean finger into the vagina. There may be days during your cycle when you have no cervical fluid (dry days), typically a few days after your period and the days following ovulation.

•Look at the cervical fluid. Note if it has a color. Earlier in the cycle or after ovulation, cervical fluid may be yellow, white or cloudy in color. As you approach ovulation, it will typically become clearer.

•Examine the consistency. It may be sticky or tacky, but on fertile days, it is usually stretchy. You may be able to stretch the fluid between your fingers on especially fertile days, and it may appear similar to egg whites.

•Note the feel of the cervical fluid. On days when you feel wet, or the cervical fluid is slippery, you may have fertile quality cervical fluid.

•Record the color, consistency, and feel of your cervical fluid during each day of your cycle. Note the day when you experienced the largest amount of slippery, clear, stretchy cervical fluid. This is your day of peak fertility. If you are tracking your temperature, you can add cervical fluid information to your existing chart.

Sample Charting

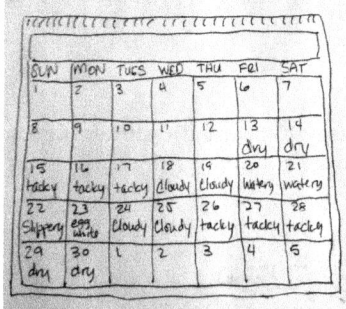

Record your basal body temperature.

Basal body temperature (BBT) is your temperature at rest. The hormone changes that occur during the menstrual cycle affect a woman's BBT. There is a slight dip in BBT immediately preceding ovulation and then a rise in temperature after ovulation that lasts throughout the luteal phase. BBT can help you identify when you ovulate during each cycle, but viewed alone, will not show you your fertile days preceding ovulation.

•Get a thermometer that will measure temperature to a tenth of a degree, a chart for recording your temperature, and a pen or pencil. Place them on your nightstand or in another location you can reach each morning without getting out of bed.

•Take your temperature each morning immediately after waking. Since BBT is the temperature of your body at rest, taking your temperature after you wake is best.

•Write down your BBT each morning on your chart. You can use a chart especially for recording fertility signs or just record the information on a piece of paper including spaces for the date, cycle day and BBT. Note any changes to your routine since illness, lack of sleep, and even using an electric blanket can all affect your BBT.

•Graph your BBT readings to see most clearly when your temperature rises during your cycle. The temperature spike is caused by the progesterone produced by the corpus luteum, and it signals that ovulation has occurred.

If you start moving will give you an inaccurate reading. Thyroid issues may throw this off so if this process seems to not be working, it's worth going to your doctor and having some thyroid labs done.

Observe changes to the cervix

The cervix will change its position during the menstrual cycle, which can help you identify when you are ovulating.

•Wash your hands.

•Insert your middle finger into the vaginal opening until you can feel your cervix.

•Note the position of the cervix, how it feels, whether or not it is wet, and how open or closed it feels. During the first few days after menstruation and the days following ovulation, the cervix is typically lower, closed, drier, and will feel firm, like the tip of your nose. During fertile days, the cervix will move up higher, be open, wet and soft.

Physical symptoms

Look for additional ovulation signs. Some women experience other physical signals that they are ovulating that can help them pinpoint when ovulation occurs during their menstrual cycles.

•Note any 1-sided pain in the lower abdomen towards the middle of your cycle. Some women experience some pain or cramping when the egg is released from 1 of the ovaries. If you have a longer menstrual cycle, ovulation should typically be 12 to 16 days from the last day of your cycle.

•Look for spotting around ovulation. This can be a sign of ovulation.

•Note any additional breast tenderness during your cycle. Although some women experience this as a symptom of premenstrual syndrome, others may experience tenderness during ovulation.

Okay, so last but not least make sure that you are having sex the days before, during and after ovulation, but relax. Don't make this a stressful time. Enjoy your relationship and relax knowing that you are on track for the first time in your baby making process. The last thing is you need to feel anxious or stressed and throw the balance off.

Supplements to ensure hormone balance, fertility and a healthy baby

[]Natural Progesterone

[]Balance Repair

[]Ultra Balance

[]Metabolic Support

[]Methyl-folate

Natural Progesterone

We have already discussed the use of the natural progesterone. Natural progesterone will also treat the symptoms of polycystic ovarian syndrome, endometriosis, irregular menstrual cycles, and all they symptoms associated with low progesterone, but most importantly, INFERTILITY.

Once you become pregnant you will want to continue the progesterone cream at a ½ dropper for the first three months to ensure enough progesterone until the pregnancy itself starts making enough progesterone. This will prevent miscarriages.

Balance Repair

This is a special blend of vital nutrients designed to relieve hormone imbalance due to excess estrogen-related issues and progesterone deficiency. This unique formula features natural selective estrogen receptor modulators (SERMs) and L-5-methyltetrahydrofolate to support multiple aspects of estrogen metabolism.

Designed to relieve common symptoms related to PMS, such as cramping, irritability, and breast tenderness.

May support breast health by promoting the hydroxylation and methylation of the "wrong kinds" of estrogen.

Provides natural selective estrogen receptor modulators (SERMs) to lessen the impact of the more potent forms of estrogen. This is the way we manipulate the conversion processes that lead to excess estrogen and not enough progesterone.

Supplies L-5-methyltetrahydrofolate, providing an advantage for those with genetic variations in folate metabolism.

Ultra Balance

This is a special blend of pro-biotics targeted Support for Feminine Health and helps restore the obliterated flora from all the issues that lead to Leaky Gut as previously discussed. This special blend has L. rhamnosus GR-1® and L. reuteri RC-14® strains.

Ultra Balance is a unique blend of probiotics taken orally to help maintain a healthy intestinal and vaginal micro-flora and support urogenital health. Healthy intestinal and vaginal micro-flora (or "friendly" bacteria) are important for women's health and well-being. But most probiotic products aren't specifically formulated to support feminine health. It's the one probiotic formula every woman should know about. The safety and efficacy of this probiotic combination for women's health is supported by more than 20 years of laboratory research and 10 years of clinical evaluation.

• In a randomized, placebo-controlled study of 64 healthy women, culture findings confirmed a significant increase in vaginal lactobacilli at days 28 and 60.*

• In a randomized, double-blind, multicenter, placebo-controlled trial of 544 subjects, restitution to healthy vaginal micro-biota was reported in 61.5% of the probiotic group.

• Effective dose in just one capsule taken orally daily

Metabolic Support

5 main ingredients to support a healthy metabolism

-Omega-3 for combating inflammation and healthy fats help balance out unhealthy fats. Omega-3 are very important for the baby's developing brain

-Iodine to help with thyroid function and iodine is essential for the baby to prevent thyroid issues like goiter and cretinism.

Methyl-folate more about this under the what you need to know to prevent birth defects section, but...:

-Methyl folate helps clear unhealthy forms of estrogen through the liver and helps eliminate toxins. Prevents build up of homocystine which can cause inflammation in the blood vessels and predispose mom to having miscarriages.

-Methyl-B12 an essential vitamin in metabolism and maintaining a healthy weight and keep energy levels up so you can chase that toddler that your baby will soon be.

-Magnesium to help with insulin sensitivity issues, most commonly found in PCOS and other fertility issues. Keeps the bowels moving and healthy and is a smooth muscle relaxer to help naturally control blood pressure should that be an issue at any point. High blood pressure in pregnancy can lead to pregnancy loss.

Maintaining a healthy pregnancy

There are many things you need to know once you get pregnant with our plan. You want a smooth pregnancy and a healthy baby or you probably wouldn't pursue this path if you thought there was a good chance that something significant could go wrong.

Well if you don't use the progesterone cream and get the right nutrients there is chance that something could go wrong.

I want to focus in this chapter on Methyl-folate, a B vitamin that is critical for you to know about. But first I'm going to tell you a little story about what I think went very wrong.

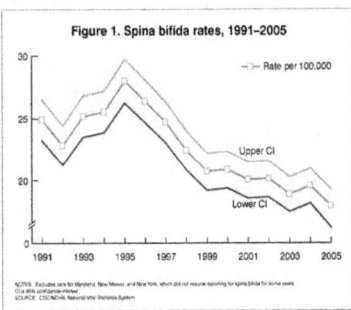

Figure 1. Spina bifida rates, 1991-2005

Our food supply changed in the 1990's. Junk food was cheaper than "real food" and we traded our vegetables for fast food. We saw an increase in spina bifida (birth defect of the spinal column and brain problems). The government began fortification as they realized from the scientists that there was a folate deficiency.

The critical B vitamin for brain development among many other functions. It was cheap to produce folic acid, so they thought it was the same thing and started putting folic acid in all the supplements and fortifying the food.

We did see a decrease in spina bifida but the problem is that a large part of the population (some studies show up to 50-70%) have a genetic defect and can't metabolize or methylate the folic acid, which can accumulate as homocysteine and cause many other problems and issues including infertility and miscarriages. In the baby it can cause autism, attention deficit disorder and later in life can lead to autoimmune disease, diabetes, sleep disorders and hormone imbalances which can lead to obesity.

I cannot stress enough that we get plenty of methyl-folate to counterbalance the effects of the folic acid that is in everything.

MTHFR, along with other gene mutations and heredity factors, can present special problems in pregnancy and reproduction. This is not to say that if you have these mutations you should be alarmed; many women with MTHFR mutations have multiple successful pregnancies before they even find out that they have these mutations. But if you're already aware of your genetic status, it would be highly beneficial to take special precautions to ensure a successful pregnancy and healthy baby (and I think testing for every person is important). I myself am currently dealing with these issues. After a miscarriage at the end prior difficulty conceiving it was a passion of mine to understand the implications of this genetic defect.

MTHFR gene mutations can create many of the same problems in pregnant women as they can in non-pregnant people. Pregnancy does, however, amplify some of the risks and effects.

Pregnant women are more prone to blood clots, for example, which are generally a risk when a person has elevated homocysteine. As we know, excess homocysteine is a common side effect of MTHFR mutations. High homocysteine can also cause pre-eclampsia and miscarriage. It is important to note also that, according to leading MTHFR researcher Dr. Ben Lynch, it isn't enough to just look at homocysteine levels when dealing with pregnancy complications and loss.

Sometimes a patient may not have an elevated serum homocysteine level, but still may have issues due to MTHFR. MTHFR mutations must be identified and addressed in order to achieve optimal results. Untreated MTHFR also puts women at a higher risk of postpartum depression.

A father's folate status and diet have been found to be Important in preventing birth defects and other diseases in offspring. So be sure he's taking methyl-folate as well and getting the proper nutrition prior to conception.

It is important to remember that MTHFR gene mutations are inherited. Therefore, depending on what mutations are present in the mother and father, the fetus is likely to inherit MTHFR in some form. The baby can inherit problems in its own DNA, which present symptoms, and can also suffer from the nutritional deficiencies of the mother that are caused by her gene mutations. The most common problem is the risk of neural tube defects because of the mother's inability to convert folic acid into l-methyl-folate.

Interesting most women take lots of folic acid thinking they are helping prevent defects. And moreover it's really scary because most all prenatal vitamins have lots of folic acid. This just blocks a person with MTHFR's ability to absorb and assimilate natural folate and methy-folate. It is a major failing of current widespread prenatal advice that more women are not aware of the problems of folic acid for so many members of the population. A lack of folate and/or B12 can cause everything from spina bifida to anencephaly to Down's syndrome. Elevated homocysteine can cause low birth weight and premature birth.

There are also additional risks once the baby is born, which makes testing for methylation gene defects important. MTHFR has been linked to congenital heart disease, autism, ADD/ADHD and a host of other illnesses. It's possible to use epigenetics to bypass the harmful effects of these mutations by taking plenty of methyl folate. Ensuring proper methylation in a baby will prevent impaired immunity and virus and heavy metal accumulation from birth. This is essential component to preventing autism and other serious health conditions.

It is especially important to avoid folic acid, which is the synthetic form of folate, if you and/or your baby has MTHFR gene mutations. This does not mean that you shouldn't consume folate. Synthetic folic acid cannot be converted properly to methyl-folate and blocks the folate receptors in people with MTHFR.

Our supplements have methyl-folate so if you are using our program you will be covered in this regard.

Egg quality can also be an issue for women with MTHFR. This is not to say that MTHFR has a direct negative impact on egg quality, but people with untreated MTHFR often have other chronic conditions that affect them. These things can cause problems with egg quality. New research has determined that the father's MTHFR status can also play a role. MTHFR has an effect on fetal viability and can also be a contributing factor to stillbirth. So if you are suffering from infertility or miscarriages, it is important to be tested for MTHFR and other genetic problems, and be sure that you are tested correctly.

The good news is that there is a lot that you can do to ensure healthy outcomes for you and your family when trying to become pregnant. The first thing will be to ensure that you and your partner are methylating properly and receiving the correct nutritional support. Be wary of any prenatal vitamins that have folic acid. Our supplements should have everything that you need.

Getting your hormones back under control after childbirth

One of the biggest complications after childbirth. Progesterone declines once the baby is born so you may want to resume the cycled progesterone regimen for at least a few months after the baby comes and continue taking our supplement regimen. Continue your exercise and eating healthy.

Breast feeding is the best way to get your body back into shape. It burns about 200 calories every time you breast feed. So now you know how to get healthy and stay healthy. I wish you the best on your journey and hope you are holding your new baby very soon.

Please email me and send me those pictures of your new baby. I always tease my patients that they have to name their baby after me. I'm only teasing but I love the thought of a lot of little Tammy's running around from our plan.

Love your baby. Embrace every day and know that I am thrilled for not only your new bundle of joy but your journey to sustainable balanced hormones and health and wellness for years to come.

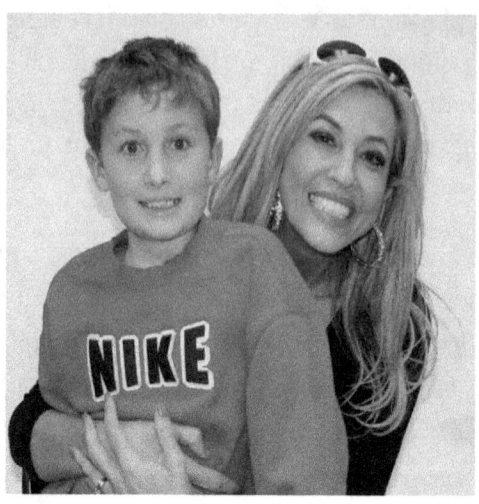

Dr. Tammy has struggled with many hormone issues including infertility and miscarriages. She was finally able to become pregnant and now is shown here with her 10 year old son. She has spent many years cultivating a culture of accountability in patients. She has motivated and mentored many in the ways of improving their own health one healthy decision at a time.

Born and raised in a small town in Arkansas and pursuing her training all throughout the U.S., she is grounded and in tune with the simple to the sophisticated when it comes to educating her patients. Her extensive work and educational background lends to her non-traditional physician approach. She went beyond attaining a bachelor's degree in biology to pursing her master's degree in public health. While doing this, she began teaching and discovered a passion for educating as a means to spawn greatness and discovery in others. She then attended 4 years of medical school at Kansas City University of Medicine and Biosciences plus an additional year at Truman Medical Center as a Pathology fellow teaching and learning about the basics of human processes. Her goal was to integrate all these experiences, so she could be the best family physician and health educator/mentor possible. She did her residency in Tallahassee, Florida. She is currently a board certified family practice physician licensed to practice in the State of Arkansas.

She has done award-winning research in multiple areas including education, cancer, and biologic hormone processes. She has focused additional emphasis on programs promoting wellness and

and preventive care. She offers her patients a unique approach to medicine by bringing an extensive education, a desire to help others, and a genuine desire to make the medical experience a positive one for all patients. Oh, and she brings a BIG SMILE! Those who know her will confirm she loves enlightening, educating, and empowering others to pursue healthy lifestyles. She has spent the past few years transforming into everything she recommends. She definitely practices what she preaches!